Becoming Mindful

Integrating Mindfulness Into Your Psychiatric Practice

Becoming Mindful

Integrating Mindfulness Into Your Psychiatric Practice

Edited by

Erin Zerbo, M.D.
Alan Schlechter, M.D.
Seema Desai, M.D.
Petros Levounis, M.D., M.A.

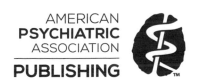

AMERICAN
PSYCHIATRIC
ASSOCIATION
PUBLISHING

Note: The authors have worked to ensure that all information in this book is accurate at the time of publication and consistent with general psychiatric and medical standards, and that information concerning drug dosages, schedules, and routes of administration is accurate at the time of publication and consistent with standards set by the U.S. Food and Drug Administration and the general medical community. As medical research and practice continue to advance, however, therapeutic standards may change. Moreover, specific situations may require a specific therapeutic response not included in this book. For these reasons and because human and mechanical errors sometimes occur, we recommend that readers follow the advice of physicians directly involved in their care or the care of a member of their family.

Books published by American Psychiatric Association Publishing represent the findings, conclusions, and views of the individual authors and do not necessarily represent the policies and opinions of American Psychiatric Association Publishing or the American Psychiatric Association.

If you wish to buy 50 or more copies of the same title, please go to www.appi.org/special discounts for more information.

Copyright © 2017 American Psychiatric Association Publishing

ALL RIGHTS RESERVED

First Edition

Manufactured in the United States of America on acid-free paper

20   19   18   17   16   5   4   3   2   1

American Psychiatric Association Publishing
1000 Wilson Boulevard
Arlington, VA 22209-3901
www.appi.org

Library of Congress Cataloging-in-Publication Data
Names: Zerbo, Erin, 1981– editor. | Schlechter, Alan, 1975– editor. | Desai, Seema, 1978– editor. | Levounis, Petros, editor. | American Psychiatric Association Publishing, issuing body.

Title: Becoming mindful : integrating mindfulness into your psychiatric practice / [edited] by Erin Zerbo, Alan Schlechter, Seema Desai, Petros Levounis.

Description: First edition. | Arlington, Virginia : American Psychiatric Association Publishing, [2017] | Includes bibliographical references and index.

Identifiers: LCCN 2016029729 (print) | LCCN 2016030901 (ebook) | ISBN 9781615370757 (pb : alk. paper) | ISBN 9781615371112

Subjects: | MESH: Mindfulness—methods | Self Care—methods | Mental Disorders—therapy

Classification: LCC RC454 (print) | LCC RC454 (ebook) | NLM WM 425.5.C6 | DDC 616.89—dc23

LC record available at https://lccn.loc.gov/2016029729

British Library Cataloguing in Publication Data
A CIP record is available from the British Library.

Contents

Contributors vii

Foreword xi

Preface xiii

1 What Is Mindfulness?
A HISTORY OF MINDFULNESS AND MEDITATION 1
Kacy Richmond, M.D.
Erin Zerbo, M.D.
Petros Levounis, M.D., M.A.

2 Plasticity and Integration
THE NEUROSCIENCE OF MINDFULNESS 9
Joseph Loizzo, M.D., Ph.D.

3 The Practice of Mindfulness 25
Kayleigh Pleas, MAPP
Cory Muscara, MAPP

4 Practice What You Preach
THE MINDFUL CLINICIAN 45
Rebecca Hedrick, M.D.
Andrea Brandon, M.D.
Seema Desai, M.D.

5 Mindfulness in Practice
INCORPORATING MINDFULNESS
INSIDE AND OUTSIDE OF SESSIONS 61
Jonathan Kaplan, Ph.D.
Doris F. Chang, Ph.D.

6 Mindfulness as an Intervention
in the Treatment of Psychopathology 79
Sarah Zoogman, Ph.D.
Elizabeth Foskolos, M.A.
Eleni Vousoura, Ph.D.

7 Finding Wellness Through
Mindfulness and Meditation
THE GROWING FIELDS OF POSITIVE PSYCHOLOGY
AND PSYCHIATRY 103
Cory Muscara, MAPP
Abigail Mengers, MAPP
Alan Schlechter, M.D.

8 Promoting Mindfulness
in Children and Adolescents 121
Mari Kurahashi, M.D., M.P.H.

9 Mindfulness-Based Interventions
for Substance Use Disorder Treatment 135
Allison K. Ungar, M.D.
Oscar G. Bukstein, M.D., M.P.H.

10 Mindful Eating. 147
Kerry Ellen Wangen, M.D., Ph.D.

11 Mindfulness and Technology 163
Matthew Diamond, M.D., Ph.D.
Patricia Zheng, M.D.
Sarah Zoogman, Ph.D.

Appendix A
AUDIO GUIDED MEDITATIONS 181

Appendix B
MINDFULNESS RESOURCES. 183

Index 187

Contributors

Andrea Brandon, M.D.
Clinical Instructor of Psychiatry, New York University School of Medicine, New York, New York

Oscar G. Bukstein, M.D., M.P.H.
Associate Psychiatrist-in-Chief and Vice Chair of Psychiatry, Boston Children's Hospital, Boston, Massachusetts

Doris F. Chang, Ph.D.
Associate Professor and Director of Clinical Training, Department of Psychology, New School for Social Research, New York, New York

Catherine C. Crone, M.D.
Associate Professor of Psychiatry, George Washington University Medical Center, Washington, D.C.; Vice Chair, Department of Psychiatry, Inova Fairfax Hospital, Falls Church, Virginia; Clinical Professor of Psychiatry, Virginia Commonwealth University School of Medicine, Northern Virginia Branch, Fairfax, Virginia

Seema Desai, M.D.
Clinical Assistant Professor of Psychiatry, New York University School of Medicine, New York, New York

Matthew Diamond, M.D., Ph.D.
Clinical Instructor, Rusk Institute of Rehabilitation Medicine, New York University School of Medicine, New York, New York

Andrea F. DiMartini, M.D.
Professor of Psychiatry and of Surgery, Western Psychiatric Institute; Consultation Liaison to the Liver Transplant Program, Starzl Transplant Institute, University of Pittsburgh Medical Center, Pittsburgh, Pennsylvania

Marian Fireman, M.D.
Clinical Professor of Psychiatry, Oregon Health & Science University, Portland, Oregon

Elizabeth Foskolos, M.A.
Ph.D. Candidate, First Department of Psychiatry, Eginition Hospital, University of Athens, Athens, Greece

Rebecca Hedrick, M.D.
Assistant Clinical Professor of Psychiatry and Associate Director, Consultation Liaison Service, Cedars-Sinai Medical Center, Los Angeles, California

Jonathan Kaplan, Ph.D.
Director and Psychologist, SoHo CBT + Mindfulness Center, New York, New York

Mari Kurahashi, M.D., M.P.H.
Clinical Instructor, Division of Child and Adolescent Psychiatry, Stanford School of Medicine, Stanford, California

Petros Levounis, M.D., M.A.
Professor and Chair, Department of Psychiatry, Rutgers New Jersey Medical School; Chief of Service, University Hospital, Newark, New Jersey

Joseph Loizzo, M.D., Ph.D.
Assistant Professor of Psychiatry, Weill Cornell Center for Integrative Medicine; Founder and Director, Nalanda Institute for Contemplative Science, New York, New York

Abigail Mengers, MAPP
Teaching Assistant, Child and Adolescent Minor in Mental Health, New York University, New York, New York

Cory Muscara, MAPP
Mindfulness Instructor, Long Island Center for Mindfulness, and Faculty, Columbia Teachers College, New York, New York; Faculty, Master of Applied Positive Psychology, University of Pennsylvania, Philadelphia, Pennsylvania

Kayleigh Pleas, MAPP
Wellness Coach and Yoga Yeacher, New York, New York

Kacy Richmond, M.D.
Resident Physician, Department of Psychiatry, University of New Mexico
Health Sciences Center, Albuquerque, New Mexico

Alan Schlechter, M.D.
Director, Bellevue Child and Adolescent Outpatient Psychiatry Clinic; Clinical
Assistant Professor of Child and Adolescent Psychiatry, New York University
School of Medicine, New York, New York

Allison K. Ungar, M.D.
Clinical Assistant Professor of Psychiatry, NYU Langone School of Medicine;
Staff Psychiatrist, VA NY Harbor Healthcare System, New York, New York

Eleni Vousoura, Ph.D.
Associate Professor of Psychology, American College of Greece-Deree; Scientific Collaborator, First Department of Psychiatry, Eginition Hospital, University of Athens, Athens, Greece

Kerry Ellen Wangen, M.D., Ph.D.
Staff Psychiatrist, Program for Traumatic Stress/PTSD, Long Beach VA, Long
Beach, California

Erin Zerbo, M.D.
Assistant Professor, Department of Psychiatry, Rutgers New Jersey Medical
School

Patricia Zheng, M.D.
Resident Physician, Department of Orthopaedic Surgery, Division of Physical
Medicine and Rehabilitation, Stanford University, Stanford, California

Sarah Zoogman, Ph.D.
Researcher, Department of Counseling and Clinical Psychology, Teachers College, Columbia University, New York, New York

Disclosure of Interests

The following contributors to this book have indicated a financial interest in or other affiliation with a commercial supporter, a manufacturer of a commercial product, a provider of a commercial service, a nongovernmental organization, and/or a government agency, as listed below:

Oscar G. Bukstein, M.D., M.P.H.   Royalties: Routledge Press, Wolters-Kluwer.

Matthew Diamond, M.D., Ph.D.   Misfit Inc. (a company that makes wearable and smart home devices to promote wellness, a wholly owned subsidiary of Fossil Group): employee compensation, equity shares, patent authorship, travel funds. Consumer Technology Association (a consumer technology trade organization that spreads awareness about the impact of consumer technology and creates technical standards as an ANSI-accredited body): membership on the Health and Fitness Technology Division Board, membership on the Board of Industry Leaders, membership on the Technology and Standards Council, chairmanship of the Health and Fitness Technology and Standards Committee, travel funds. National Sleep Foundation (a nonprofit organization aimed at improving public health and safety by achieving an increased understanding of sleep and sleep disorders and supporting sleep-related education, research, and advocacy): membership on the Sleep Technology Council. Center for Personalized Health Monitoring, University of Massachusetts Amherst (a research, partnership, and demonstration facility within the Institute for Health Monitoring Applied Life Sciences, aimed at accelerating the commercialization of health-related technology): membership on the Industry Advisory Board. Sohn, Inc. (medical device startup company): membership on the Medical Advisory Board, equity ownership.

The following contributors to this book have no competing interests to report:

Andrea Brandon, M.D.; Seema Desai, M.D.; Elizabeth Foskolos, M.A.; Rebecca Hedrick, M.D.; Jonathan Kaplan, Ph.D.; Mari Kurahashi, M.D., M.P.H.; Petros Levounis, M.D., M.A.; Joseph Loizzo, M.D., Ph.D., Kayleigh Pleas, MAPP, Kacy Richmond, M.D.; Alan Schlechter, M.D.; Allison K. Ungar, M.D.; Eleni Vousoura, Ph.D.; Kerry Ellen Wangen, M.D., Ph.D.; Erin Zerbo, M.D.; Sarah Zoogman, Ph.D.

Foreword

IN medical school we learn about the components of the body and the direction of their influences on each other, with genes, cells, and organs leading to how the body, brain, and mind function. We now know that the mind itself can alter the structure of the brain and enhance the function of various systems in the body, improving the cardiovascular and immune systems as well as shaping the epigenetic regulatory molecules that help diminish inflammation and increasing levels of the telomerase enzyme that maintains and repairs the ends of our chromosomes. These empirically established findings are scientific fact, not wishful thinking.

If you heard of a medication that would create these hard-earned, scientifically established findings, you might invest in that product. If we replace the "c" in "medication" with a "t," we arrive at the intervention: mindfulness meditation. *Becoming Mindful* offers a magnificent overview of what it means to be mindful, how research supports the positive effects of mindfulness on both practitioner and patient health, and how you as a practitioner can learn to cultivate a more mindful life for yourself and for patients in your clinical practice. With carefully assembled chapters providing both an introduction to this exciting and important field and in-depth, special topic–focused applications, the contributors to this comprehensive yet concise volume have created a wonderful way to learn about this important aspect of health-promotion available to us all.

For professionals in medicine and other clinical fields, the knowledge and practical suggestions included in this book, grounded in science and articulated with stunning clarity and everyday utility, will be hugely beneficial to the well-being of both the reader and any patient fortunate enough to have that individual caring for them. Reading this work is a win-win experience.

Daniel J. Siegel, M.D.
Clinical Professor of Psychiatry, UCLA School of Medicine
Founding Co-Director, UCLA Mindful Awareness Research Center
Executive Director, Mindsight Institute
Author of *Mind: A Journey to the Heart of Being Human* and other
texts, including *Pocket Guide to Interpersonal Neurobiology, The Developing
Mind, The Mindful Brain, The Mindful Therapist, Brainstorm,* and *Mindsight*

Preface

THIS is a selfish book.

The little volume on mindfulness that you are holding in your hands will help you develop your own mindfulness practices, both for yourself and for your patients. At the same time, we, the authors, greatly improved ourselves as psychiatrists (*and* as garden variety human beings) by writing it.

Mindfulness has made our own lives richer, has brought a sense of peace and clarity to our chaotic, busy existences, and has helped us to slow down and truly enjoy the moment. Our patients benefit as well—we are better listeners and better clinicians and are more receptive when we are in a mindful state. Above all, teaching these skills to patients is the perfect way to "pay it forward" by assisting them in expanding their own capacity for distress, improving their ability to cope, and living with greater well-being.

We have put together this book as a practical, down-to-earth guide that should be as fun to read as it was fun to write. The initial chapters introduce the concept of mindfulness, describe its history, and delve into the neuroscience behind it. But the heart of the book comes next: how to actually practice mindfulness, how to teach it to others, and how to deal with pitfalls and roadblocks that may be encountered. We have provided examples and guided meditations to ease the transition and build confidence in using these skills.

The later chapters in the book explore applications of mindfulness among the patients whom we treat: persons with various types of psychopathology, children and adolescents, and individuals with addiction. Mindfulness has become a widely used concept these days, and we wanted to showcase some of this work as well; therefore, we have also included chapters on mindful eating, the relationship between mindfulness and technology, and the growing field of positive psychiatry and psychology.

The book's primary audience is the practitioner or trainee who is interested in sharpening her or his skills in mindfulness. We hope to convince the reader that practicing mindfulness is learnable, teachable, and enjoyable—and it is only a breath away.

We would like to thank our patients, teachers, students, and colleagues at Rutgers New Jersey Medical School and New York University School of Medicine, without whom none of this would be possible. Finally, we are very thankful to our partners in crime: three husbands and one wife—Sal, Carlyn, Josh, and Lukas. Without them, remaining mindful through the long haul of writing and editing would have been enormously difficult.

Erin Zerbo, M.D.

Alan Schlechter, M.D.

Seema Desai, M.D.

Petros Levounis, M.D., M.A.

Newark, New Jersey, and New York City
Spring 2016

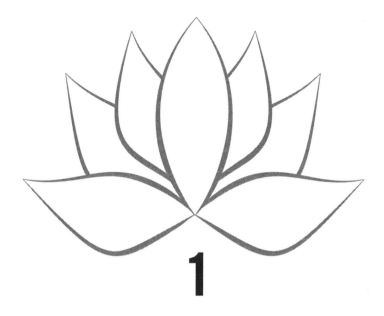

1

What Is Mindfulness?

A History of
Mindfulness and Meditation

Kacy Richmond, M.D.
Erin Zerbo, M.D.
Petros Levounis, M.D., M.A.

We have more possibilities available in each moment
than we realize.

Thich Nhat Hanh

Two THOUSAND FIVE HUNDRED years ago, in the texts of the *Satipaṭṭhāna* and *Ānāpānasati Sutras*, Buddha taught the basic principles of what we today call "mindfulness." Mindfulness is a state of mind that appreciates the flow of consciousness in real time and with acceptance. This deliberate attention to experiences as they transpire must occur without the higher-level cognitive functions that label thoughts as positive or negative and without getting trapped in any one circular or emotional thought related to the past or future (Gunaratana 2002). Mindfulness is often defined as "sustained present moment awareness," a state that allows all thoughts to arise and fall away while one attends to them "behind the screen" with curiosity and a nonjudgmental attitude (Kabat-Zinn 2003).

This awareness does not come naturally to most people. In a sage observation of contemporary obstacles to the practice of mindfulness, Jon Kabat-Zinn (2003) writes, "Perhaps [mindfulness] is only strange in a society that persists in devaluating the present moment in favor of perpetual distraction, self-absorption, and addiction to a feeling of 'progress'" (p. 148). Given the challenges to its adoption, mindfulness is typically cultivated in a daily solo meditation practice or in group retreats.

Mindfulness meditation is also called *insight meditation*, or *vipassanā bhāvanā* in the Pali language (Gunaratana 2002). Training one's mind to adopt the flexible mental state that attends to all thoughts clearly while reserving judgment is thought to lead to a more accurate understanding of reality and an improved ability to cope with difficult experiences (Siegel et al. 2009). In his brilliant and readable book *Mindfulness in Plain English*, Gunaratana (2002) suggests that one interpretation of *appamada*, a Pali word for "mindfulness," is the nonexistence of madness or total sanity, a state that may be achieved through the practice of willfully directing one's attention to present experiences.

In the past 35 years, mindfulness has exploded in popularity thanks to influential American teachers such as Jon Kabat-Zinn; scientific studies that attest to its effectiveness in reducing stress; and its widespread espousal by leaders in business, education, medicine, and the media. Watching Anderson Cooper with electrodes on his head to measure mindfulness-induced electroencephalographic changes in the December 14, 2014, episode of *60 Minutes*, one might not guess that the mindfulness tradition in the Western world had a revolutionary start.

The modern roots of the mindfulness movement come from the Theravāda branch of Buddhism and date back to eighteenth-century Burma, when a monk named Medawi wrote meditation manuals that encouraged monks to return to the practice during a time when interest in Buddha's teachings had dwindled (Sharf 2015). According to Buddhist scholar Robert Sharf (2015), Burmese teachers in the tradition of Medawi influenced Mahasi Sayadaw (1904–1982), the monk who radically transformed the way *vipassanā* meditation was practiced. Mahasi Sayadaw's progressive and egalitarian meditation method consisted of concentrating on what was happening at the present moment through the observation of bodily sensations. His technique did not require previous experience, religious worship, knowledge of Buddhism, or an ascetic lifestyle (Fronsdal 1998). The technique also had no hierarchy or ritual as in traditional meditation practices, and it could be learned in a short amount of time. It spread rapidly and became popular in East Asia and the West (Fronsdal 1998).

The *vipassanā* movement started by Mahasi Sayadaw came to include most of the modern Western Buddhist teachers. As Sharf (2015) recounts, Mahasi Sayadaw's student Nyanaponika Thera, a German who fled to Sri Lanka from the Nazis, is credited with the invention of the term *bare attention* in his 1954 book *The Heart of Buddhist Meditation*. In 1976, Sharon Salzberg, Jack Kornfield, and Joseph Goldstein cofounded the Insight Meditation Society (IMS) in Massachusetts after studying in Southeast Asia with master *vipassanā* teachers, both monastic and lay. The IMS remains the most vital *vipassanā* meditation center in the West, leading days-long retreats and training teachers (Fronsdal 1998). Other powerful early figures in American mindfulness include Ruth Denison, who led the first women's Buddhist meditation retreat in the United States in the 1970s; Gil Fronsdal, whose audio podcasts on Buddhist teachings are widely downloaded; and Tara Brach, who is best known for her compassionate approach to healing with mindfulness.

Jon Kabat-Zinn recognized the potential for mindfulness meditation to serve as a method to help people manage pain and suffering. In 1979, he created the 8-week Mindfulness-Based Stress Reduction (MBSR) program at the University of Massachusetts Medical Center. By branding mindfulness as a stress-reduction technique, Kabat-Zinn intended to make the program free from any mention of Buddhism that could be off-putting for patients already entrenched in their own religious ideas (Harrington and Dunne 2015). This clearly had its origin in Mahasi Sayadaw's secular mid-twentieth-century teachings. Kabat-Zinn's program has proven hugely successful. Hundreds of similar programs now exist across the United States, and the treatment has shown effectiveness for anxiety and depression. MBSR also set the stage for other mindfulness-based therapies that followed, including mindfulness-based cognitive therapy, dialectical behavior therapy, and acceptance and commitment therapy. Interest in mindfulness-based therapies has intensified in recent years, and there has been a growing demand for its use in corporations, the military, and a variety of other professional settings (Harrington and Dunne 2015).

Before the involvement of American teachers in the insight meditation movement of the 1970s, Western audiences first became familiar with Buddhist meditation in the 1950s through the efforts of the charismatic Japanese teacher of Zen, Daisetz Teitaro Suzuki (1870–1966) (McCown et al. 2010). Zen meditation is practiced by focusing exclusively on sitting with an empty mind or by concentrating on a paradoxical question to force the mind into an intuitive understanding of reality (Gunaratana 2002). Suzuki's writings about Zen inspired not only psychotherapists such as Carl Jung (who wrote an introduction to one of Suzuki's books) and Erich Fromm but also Beat poets such as Allen Ginsberg. The characters in Jack Kerouac's 1958 novel *The Dharma Bums* search for meaning through Zen spirituality (McCown et al. 2010).

Zen Buddhism continues to attract devoted followers in the United States, but starting in the 1960s and 1970s, national attention turned to a new form of mysticism: Transcendental Meditation (TM; McCown et al. 2010). The Hindu technique, which was popularized by Maharishi Mahesh Yogi from India, focused on the repetition of a mantra chosen specifically for the meditator. After the Beatles met the Maharishi in the 1960s and adopted him as their spiritual guide, other celebrities followed suit (McCown et al. 2010). Herbert Benson published the first studies of transcendental meditators in the 1970s (Bleich and Boro 1977). He documented encephalographic changes and decreases in heart rate, oxygen consumption, respiratory rate, and arterial blood lactate and termed these effects the "relaxation response." This and other scientific studies that followed challenged the Western notion of mind-body separation and catapulted TM to multinational fame (Harrington and Dunne 2015). Today, there is no consensus on the beneficial effects of TM, and research attention has shifted away from TM to mindfulness meditation. Chapter 2, "Plasticity and Integration," provides an overview of the latest in the growing body of research literature on mindfulness.

Unlike prayer, Zen meditation, and TM, mindfulness meditation does not call for concentration on one object to the exclusion of all others (Gunaratana 2002). Through its focus on individual practice that does not require ritual or an extensive philosophical foundation, mindfulness is also less exclusive, less demanding, and more accessible than the forms of meditation that have preceded it (Sharf 2015). Mindfulness lacks a charismatic leader and is recognized for its egalitarianism; it was the first of the popular Buddhist schools of thought to have women teachers (McCown et al. 2010).

This aim of this book is to illustrate the practical value and accessibility of mindfulness meditation for the patient as well as for the clinician. Researcher Dan Siegel (2007) suggests that mindfulness engenders compassion: the midline prefrontal areas of the brain that change as a result of mindfulness meditation are also the areas that are active when a person is empathizing with others, regulating his or her emotions, paying attention, and engaging in moral reasoning (the activities of an effective clinician). Buddhist teacher Joseph Goldstein (2013) makes a compelling argument that everyone stands to benefit from improving his or her life of the mind:

> One of the most important foundational understandings of the Buddhist teachings has to do with…the truth of karma, which means that our actions…of our body or our speech or our mind bring results…. What we do, how we act, the way we speak has an effect not only on other people, but on our own minds. We are creating, moment to moment, our own inner mental environment. This is the environment we inhabit in our lives. When we understand this, we begin to take more responsibility for our actions, for our speech, for our thoughts, what we choose to give energy to, what we choose to let go of, because we realize that our own happiness depends on this awareness…. Which qualities of mind are we actually cultivating?

Because mindfulness enhances well-being, in the middle part of this book (Chapters 3–7), we focus on developing the clinician's own practice of mindfulness in addition to learning how to use mindfulness with patients. We provide detailed instructions and delve into challenges that people—both clinicians and patients—often face when they begin to practice mindfulness. There are a multitude of applications for mindfulness in clinical populations with psychopathology, and this is explored in depth in Chapter 6, "Mindfulness as an Intervention in the Treatment of Psychopathology."

What can be accomplished with mindfulness, besides self-improvement? In the latter chapters of this book (Chapters 8–11), we explore selected special topics in mindfulness and ways it can be used to help particular patients. These subspecialty areas are mindfulness in youth populations (Chapter 8), the use of mindfulness among individuals with addiction (Chapter 9), mindful eating (Chapter 10), and mindfulness as it relates to technology (Chapter 11). These areas were chosen for their broad applicability.

In Appendix A, the reader will find two guided audio meditations that were recorded specifically for this book; they are for use in the office or at home. Appendix B contains a list of resources on mindfulness, including phone applications for use in daily meditation practice; lists of retreat centers, videos, and podcasts; and suggestions for further reading.

The use of mindfulness is growing by leaps and bounds in many disparate fields, and this is clearly due to its charm—it is effective, easy to use, and portable. We hope that this book is a helpful start for the clinician to dive in, right in her or his own office.

References

Bleich HL, Boro ES: Systemic hypertension and the relaxation response. N Engl J Med 296(20):1152–1156, 1977 323702

Fronsdal G: Insight meditation in the United States: life, liberty, and the pursuit of happiness, in The Faces of Buddhism in America. Edited by Prebish CS, Tanaka KK. Berkeley, University of California Press, 1998, pp 163–182

Goldstein J: Buddhism: The Essential Points (video file). April 23, 2013. Available at: https://www.youtube.com/watch?v=LgkBnMu_cdM. Accessed January 18, 2016.

Gunaratana H: Mindfulness in Plain English. Boston, MA, Wisdom Publications, 2002

Harrington A, Dunne JD: When mindfulness is therapy: ethical qualms, historical perspectives. Am Psychol 70(7):621–631, 2015 26436312

Kabat-Zinn J: Mindfulness-based interventions in context: past, present, and future. Clin Psychol Sci Pract 10(2):144–156, 2003

McCown D, Reibel D, Micozzi MS: Teaching Mindfulness: A Practical Guide for Clinicians and Educators. New York, NY, Springer, 2010

Sharf RH: Is mindfulness Buddhist? (and why it matters). Transcult Psychiatry 52(4):470–484, 2015 25361692

Siegel DJ: Mindfulness training and neural integration: differentiation of distinct streams of awareness and the cultivation of well-being. Soc Cogn Affect Neurosci 2(4):259–263, 2007

Siegel RD, Germer CK, Olendzki A: Mindfulness: what is it? where did it come from? in Handbook of Mindfulness. Edited by Didonna F. New York, Springer, 2009, pp 17–35

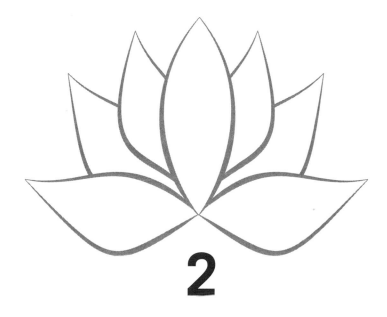

2

Plasticity and Integration

The Neuroscience of Mindfulness

Joseph Loizzo, M.D., Ph.D.

Mental activities, such as purposely paying attention to the present moment, actually stimulate the brain to become active in specific ways that then promote the growth of integrative regions. These neuroplastic changes…help us see the link between mindful awareness and the creation of well-being.

Daniel Siegel, *The Mindful Brain*

THE GROWING ROLE of mindfulness in psychiatry dates to the beginnings of meditation research. As soon as Benson and Kabat-Zinn evolved the first evidence-based paradigms for the clinical use of meditation—the relaxation response (Beary and Benson 1974) and Mindfulness-Based Stress Reduction (MBSR) (Kabat-Zinn 1982)—they began studying the application of these methods in mental health. The results of the first pilot studies in anxiety (Benson et al. 1978) were promising enough to encourage the development of clinical paradigms tailored for mental health. Early paradigms used mindfulness in treatment-resistant conditions such as borderline personality (Linehan et al. 1991) and recurrent depression (Teasdale et al. 1995). Because studies of Linehan's Dialectical Behavior Therapy (DBT) and Teasdale's Mindfulness-Based Cognitive Therapy (MBCT) showed reductions in self-injurious behavior and depression relapse, mindfulness was applied to other conditions, and interest in it as an adjunct in mental health grew (Baer 2003).

Meanwhile, understanding of the neural mechanisms of mindfulness grew exponentially. In my first review (Loizzo 2000), I proposed that meditation shares a common mechanism with psychotherapy, combining two elements: the reduction of stress and the enrichment of learning. The most common conditions treated in psychiatry have been linked to "wear and tear" on the brain, caused by overexposure to stress hormones and inflammatory cytokines. In contrast to the adaptive responses to normal challenges called *allostasis*, the syndrome of "wear and tear" caused by chronic stress and trauma has been described as *allostatic load/overload*. Around the same time, others reported a seemingly contradictory finding: under persistent positive stimulation, the brain underwent tissue growth, repair, and regeneration. This "use it or lose it" process, now known as *neuroplasticity*, not only counterbalanced the wear and tear of stress but was linked to findings that learning and neurogenesis were enhanced in "enriched environments" (Rosenzweig and Bennett 1996).

The implications of neuroplasticity did not escape the attention of pioneers like Kandel, who made it the basis for a new paradigm in psychiatry (Kandel 1998). However, the paradigm he proposed would not be complete without another line of research. Twenty years after the stress response was described (Selye 1955), Benson introduced the idea of the relaxation response as its complement (Beary and Benson 1974). Given the binary structure of the autonomic nervous system (ANS) and the role of sympathetic activation in stress, meditation was said to elicit the relaxation response by increasing parasympathetic activation. Research on MBSR distinguished mindfulness, as "a discipline of attention," from the relaxation response (Goleman and Schwartz 1976). In contrast to relaxation alone, the effects of mindfulness were attributed to a hybrid mechanism like the one I proposed: meditation's calming function improving allostasis by reducing the stress response and its attentional function enriching learning by stimulating use-dependent plasticity (Davidson 2000).

Further studies supported the mechanistic role of neuroplasticity, linking mindfulness with electroencephalogram (EEG) patterns and structural changes consistent with increased activation, myelination, and neurogenesis (Lazar et al. 2000, 2005). One key study showed that Tibetan-trained experts were able to consciously induce EEG findings indicative of increased learning and plasticity—unprecedented trains of gamma activity and synchrony—at will (Lutz et al. 2004). More recent studies confirmed the link between meditation and neurogenesis (Hölzel et al. 2011a; Luders et al. 2009) and also linked meditation to brain connectivity (Gard et al. 2014; Jang et al. 2011). Today, meditation is seen as a missing link in conscious self-regulation, connecting mental training to the electrochemical processes of neuronal firing, epigenetic regulation of gene transcription, and new neural connectivity.

Whereas such studies have clarified how mindfulness enriches learning, related findings have revealed the other side of its mechanism and effects: conscious ANS regulation. Decades of studies of conscious breath practices have all shown some modulation of the ANS (Harinath et al. 2004). The understanding of such shifts has been expanded by more recent work on the ANS (Porges 2011). Porges explains how the myelinated "smart vagus" that evolved in mammals not only supports voluntary breathing but also helps modulate primitive vagal and sympathetic reflexes to support expanded use of higher cortical capacities for social engagement.

Another general model views meditation as an integrative practice. When attention and relaxation combine, they help shift the dissociative, reactive mode of neural processing that prevails under stress, trauma, and insecure attachment to the integrative, responsive style of processing that emerges under conditions of social safety, positive stimulation, and secure attachment (Siegel 2012). Integrative models and mindfulness converge in research on the most recently evolved brain region: the prefrontal cortex (PFC). An inventory of prefrontal functions reads like a wish list of human development: selective attention and working memory, planning and execution, emotion regulation, empathy and morality, problem solving, and body awareness. Given its intimate links with other brain regions—neocortical, limbic, subcortical, midbrain, and brain stem—the PFC is seen as the "conductor" of the neural symphony and the seat of conscious brain integration. Not surprisingly, the PFC also plays the central role in current meditation research, as seen in Vago's (2014) model of mindfulness as enhancing an integrative network based in the PFC, fostering self-awareness, self-regulation, and self-transcendence.

Mindfulness and Psychotherapy: Vertical and Lateral Integration

For decades, researchers have reflected on the similarities between mindfulness and free association. Apart from the surface resemblance between Freud's "evenly hovering attention" and descriptions of mindfulness as "unbiased awareness," these reflections raise two deeper mechanistic questions (Loizzo 2000): What level of consciousness do mindfulness and free association occupy along the spectrum from normal wakefulness to sleep or trance? Which mode of consciousness do they engage on the bimodal spectrum from abstract-analytic to embodied-sensorimotor?

EEG studies of common meditation techniques such as Transcendental Meditation and mindfulness show a pattern of gradually increasing neocortical alpha amplitude and coherence (Fenwick 1987), suggesting an initial phase of deepening introspection and calm comparable to drowsiness (Cahn and Polich 2006). However, meditators routinely stop the progression that normally leads to somnolence, and instead of generating slow theta or delta waves typical of stage 1 sleep, they produce a rise of high-frequency theta activity, consistent with increased attentiveness (Gruzelier 2009). A similar pattern of wakeful relaxation is thought to be cultivated by free association, which Freud conceived as "waking-state hypnosis" (DelMonte 1995).

The question of where mindfulness falls on the spectrum of states of consciousness relates to the theme of vertical integration. Although some dissociation between levels and states of consciousness is the default condition of the human mind-brain, it would appear that with the right methods and repeated practice, they can be reorganized into an integrated system. In fact, the level of consciousness at which insight and attention can be maintained is not fixed but instead varies with the type of practice and the level of expertise. This is evident not only from studies that show self-regulation of deeper structures with expertise (Luders et al. 2013; Lutz et al. 2008) but also from studies of virtuosos who show markers of waking state consciousness in the dream and deep sleep states (Mason et al. 1997) and of aroused consciousness in hypometabolic states resembling hibernation, estivation, and the diving state of aquatic mammals (Heller et al. 1987).

Given the increasing evidence of lateral specialization among the cerebral hemispheres, as well as among key subcortical structures such as the insula, cingulate, hippocampus, and amygdala, the second question is how meditation and psychotherapy alter hemispheric lateralization. Since Roger Sperry's studies of epileptics with surgically bisected hemispheres (Sperry 1974), evidence has mounted that the verbal-expressive left hemisphere preferentially supports analytic processing, optimistic thinking, positive affect, and approach behaviors, whereas the sensorimotor-receptive right hemisphere supports synthetic processing, worst-case thinking, aversive affect, and avoidance. This is consistent with findings that vagal activation generally dominates left hemisphere processing, whereas sympathetic activation tends to dominate on the right (Shannahoff-Khalsa 2007). The mix of moderate relaxation with heightened attention common to both meditation and psychotherapy suggests that they may share a mechanism of altering hemispheric laterality (Loizzo 2009). This mechanism has been supported by numerous findings and explained in two ways.

DelMonte (1995) suggested that a shift toward balanced dominance reduces the default dissociation between the hemispheres, offering verbal consciousness greater access to normally suppressed emotion and repressed trauma. This is consistent with findings that meditation increases the size of the corpus callosum (Luders et al. 2012), increases cortical integration (Gard et al. 2014; Luders et al. 2011), increases the activity and size of the right anterior cingulate cortex (ACC) and the right insula (Lazar et al. 2005), decreases the activation and size of the right amygdala (Hölzel et al. 2010), and increases activation in implicit learning structures such as the caudate and putamen (Tang et al. 2009).

Davidson et al. (2003) offer a complementary explanation, based on the left lateral shift in prefrontal activity in mindfulness. They attribute the enhanced emotion regulation in mindfulness to greater involvement of the left hemisphere. This finding is consistent with the clinical evidence that mindfulness helps prevent depression relapse by enhancing metacognition (Teasdale et al. 1995), as well as with findings of increased attentional flexibility and resilience in meditators (Gard et al. 2014). It also overlaps with recent clinical models of common psychopathology—anxiety, depression, trauma, attention deficit, impulse control, and addictive disorders—as a syndrome of hypofrontality: a dysregulation of limbic reactivity and subcortical impulsivity based on developmental deficits or disuse of "top-down" prefrontal regulatory centers and pathways (Menon 2011).

Both these explanations have validity, and they reflect complementary mechanisms. Increased access to normally suppressed, dissociated, or repressed material opens the way to deeper insight, corrective experience, and transformation. Higher faculties of metacognitive insight, narrative reframing, and emotion regulation are equally necessary to constructively reprocess the newly accessed material. This second general mechanism shared by meditation and psychotherapy clearly relates to the theme of lateral integration. As in vertical integration, it appears that the human mind and brain have a greater capacity for lateral integration than previously thought, especially when given rigorous methods and practice (Luders et al. 2012).

The Full Spectrum of Mindfulness: Modes of Practice, Mechanism, and Integration

Given the preceding overview, we can now analyze the full spectrum of mindfulness, its neural mechanisms, and its effects, under three main headings. After subdividing mindfulness into five distinct modes of practice, on the basis of the literature I will align the modes with one of Vago's (2014) three broad mechanisms of action—self-awareness, self-regulation, and self-transcendence—and map their effects onto three levels of integration: neocortical, limbic, and core brain. In addition, I touch on how each of the modes of practice, mechanisms of action, and levels of integration are finding their way into contemplative psychotherapy.

The five modes of mindfulness practice taught in the tradition are 1) mindfulness of the body, 2) mindfulness of sensitivity, 3) mindfulness of mindset, 4) mindfulness of mentality, and 5) loving-kindness. In the following sections, I align the practice of mindful body with the mechanism of self-awareness and the effect of neocortical integration. I align mindful sensitivity and loving-kindness with self-regulation and limbic integration. Finally, I align mindful mindset and mindful mentality with self-transcendence and core brain integration.

Mindful Body and Self-Awareness: Integrating the Neocortex

Of the five basic modes of mindfulness practice, the simplest—body mindfulness—begins by using breath as a focal point to reconnect conscious attention to the body. This practice offers an accessible, reproducible methodology for building attention and cultivating self-awareness, as proposed in Vago's (2014) first mechanism of mindfulness—self-awareness. Because all mindfulness practice exercises awareness, it is no surprise that such practice has been found to heighten attention and expand working memory, increasing activation and gray matter in executive regions such as the dorsolateral and anterior PFC (Lazar et al. 2005; Luders et al. 2009). Mindfulness has been shown to increase not only attention but also metacognitive functions such as attentional flexibility, fluid intelligence (Jha et al. 2007), resilience, global network efficiency, and network integration (Gard et al. 2014). Consistent with this expansion of metacognitive awareness, mindfulness has also been shown to enhance emotion regulation (Creswell et al. 2007) by greater activation of the orbitofrontal region of the PFC (Hölzel et al. 2011b) but not at the cost of a dissociation from sensitivity. In fact, mindfulness enhances body self-awareness, increasing the activation and size of the (right) insula, a deep neocortical region that serves as an interoceptive map or link to bodily sensations (Farb et al. 2013), and increasing the activation and size of the right thalamus (Luders et al. 2009). Likewise, mindfulness and related practices have been found to enhance perceptual sensitivity, introspective accuracy (Fox et al. 2012), and the discrimination of emotions (MacLean et al. 2010).

Among the findings linking mindfulness with neocortical self-awareness, the most intriguing relate to the impact of mindfulness on the offline processing of the default mode network. The default mode network maintains the internally generated loop of self-referential narrative and self-world imagery that fills the void when mind and brain are idling between tasks. This network functions differently in meditators and nonmeditators, with the former showing less self-referential activity not only in practice sessions but also in everyday life (Brewer et al. 2011). Mindfulness practice, however, does not lead to a detached self-awareness stuck in a pure, internal present. It opens self-awareness outward to the world, growing mirror regions and default mode network regions that support facial recognition, the self-other empathy system, and cerebellar regions involved in planning and executing intentional action (Hölzel et al. 2011b). These findings suggest that mindfulness increases self-awareness and neocortical integration by deautomatizing self-constructive processing and bringing metacognitive awareness and flexibility to default habits of identity, social recognition, and intentionality. The evidence that mindfulness practice helps expand the capacity of the neocortex for integrated social engagement is also consistent with Porges's (2011) model of ANS modulation.

Therapeutically, basic mindfulness not only is a key element in MBCT but works like free association to support dynamic psychotherapy, fostering the emergence of observing ego and insight as alternatives to self-limiting ego defenses. This neocortical mechanism may help explain why mindfulness strengthens recovery from depression and why it has been taken up as a helpful adjunct in psychodynamic practice.

Mindful Sensitivity, Kindness, and Self-Regulation: Integrating the Limbic System

The second basic mode of mindfulness practice—mindful sensitivity—focuses on the raw feelings of pleasure, pain, and neutrality that color all experiences of body, mind, and world and trigger subliminal reactivity to positive, negative, and neutral stimulation. This key practice trains the mind to anticipate and prevent sensory reactivity based on past conditioning. It also dovetails with the mindfulness-based practice of loving-kindness, which trains the mind to prevent reactive emotions, such as fear, rage, and shame, by anticipating and transforming them into proactive emotions, such as kindness, tolerance, and acceptance.

The first two modes of practice relate to Vago's (2014) second mechanism of mindfulness: self-regulation. The relevance of self-regulation to mindfulness stems from the vulnerability of the neocortex to dysregulation, based on the default self-protective structure of the human brain. The neocortex maintains its default social engagement mode—led by the PFC—only under conditions of perceived safety. Once the brain detects potential harm, it typically shifts into stress-protective mode, under the influence of the amygdala. This shift not only triggers the general stress response, with its sympathetic and hypothalamic-pituitary-adrenal axis components, but also disables the top-down regulation of the PFC and "hijacks" the neocortex. In this mode, the brain falls into a functional syndrome of hypofrontality. The damage done is compounded when the stresses are chronic, and individuals end up in states of allostatic overload, such as depression, chronic fatigue syndrome, learned helplessness, or posttraumatic stress disorder.

Mindfulness has been shown to decrease levels of anxiety and perceived stress, a finding correlated with decreased activation and gray matter in the right amygdala (Goldin et al. 2013). One mechanism for this enhanced self-regulation of "bottom-up" stress reactivity is increased activation of the ACC by regions of the PFC known to moderate fear and stress perception (Posner et al. 2007), because the ACC is the hub for top-down control of the limbic system by cognitive-emotional integration. Tang et al. (2009) found that a practice of mind-body self-regulation similar to mindfulness, in addition to heightening attention, increased ACC activation as well as heart rate variability, a measure of smart vagal activation.

Another mechanism of self-regulation in mindful sensitivity reflects the increasing emotional context provided by the hippocampus. If the amygdala is the brain's emotional alarm bell, the hippocampus serves as its emotional moderator or damper. Given its function to form and retain explicit memories, the hippocampus maps present data points onto an inner universe of spatiotemporal, social-emotional, and narrative perspective. The reference setting of the hippocampus helps contextualize raw sensory input processed in the amygdala, reframing worst-case fears in light of a broader range of personal and interpersonal experience.

In addition to mindful sensitivity, the second main mode of practice for self-regulation of the emotional brain is loving-kindness or compassion practice.

The past decade has seen a number of key findings that clarify the effectiveness and mechanisms of loving-kindness. Fredrickson et al. (2008) found that simple loving-kindness meditation—exercising and gradually expanding positive emotions toward self and others in a mindful state—enhanced a range of positive emotions, expanded well-being, and enriched social resources and relationships. More recent studies have shed light on the mechanisms of compassion training. The normal brain typically responds to seeing distressed faces with activation of the frontoparietal mirror neuron system and middle ACC, which triggers conditioned disgust activation in the anterior insula and fear reactivity in the amygdala. After brief mindful compassion training, novices' brains showed less connectivity of the PFC with the anterior insula and amygdala, more activation of PFC regulatory regions (the dorsolateral prefrontal cortex and medial orbitofrontal cortex) and the superior ACC intentional hub (Klimecki et al. 2013), and significant activation of mesolimbic reward system structures (Weng et al. 2013). These effects of kindness-compassion practice reflect a self-regulatory shift in limbic functioning from a bottom-up social-emotional stress-reactive mode to a top-down mode of positive affective self-regulation and proactive social engagement.

Clinically, the first intervention integrating mindful sensitivity and kindness practices was Linehan's DBT (Linehan et al. 1991). More recently, the study of inwardly directed kindness practice as "self-compassion" was proposed as integral to the effects of interventions such as MBSR and MBCT, suggesting the broad therapeutic potential of self-regulatory forms of mindfulness practice (Kuyken et al. 2010; Neff 2003). A second generation of interventions has developed around Tibetan methods, formulated as cognitively based compassion training (Desbordes et al. 2012) and compassion cultivation training (Klimecki et al. 2014). The most developed of these is the compassion-focused therapy formulated by Paul Gilbert (2014) on the basis of MBCT. Initial studies show that this therapy has real promise as an intervention for a range of mental and physical health issues, including treatment of depression, anxiety, and psychosis, and for smoking cessation (Leaviss and Uttley 2015). Finally, the practice of mindful sensitivity and kindness has been artfully woven into object relational approaches to psychotherapy by psychoanalysts Mark Epstein (1995) and Jeffrey Rubin (1996).

Mindfulness and Self-Transcendence: Integrating the Core Brain

The last two modes of practices—mindful mindset and mentality—are the least known modes of mindfulness because they are more challenging to teach, learn, and practice than the previous three. In mindful mindset, attention is focused on the primary process of mind, traditionally taken to mean the raw data of sense intuitions or mental impressions prior to any association with verbal concepts, symbolic images, or emotional memories. The benefits of such "upstream" access to preprocessed mind-body states have obvious relevance to the correction of conditioned associations involved in bottom-up reactivity to stress and trauma. The complement to this practice is mindful mentality. This practice, which is based on direct access to preprocessed input via mindfulness of mindset, brings unbiased awareness to the way that input is processed by conditioned associations to memory images, emotional responses, and verbal narratives. It allows a metacognitive assessment and correction of the mentality with which the input is processed, including correcting perceptual distortions, reactive emotions, and/or traumatic narratives. This set of practices presents a depth-psychological insight practice meant to support self-transcendence through the deconstruction and reconstruction of personality (Dahl et al. 2015; Davidson 2013).

The first potential mechanism for the practice of mindful mindset comes from findings that mindfulness increases activation and gray matter in core brain regions critical to sense perception and implicit learning: the caudate, putamen, and thalamus (Pickut et al. 2013; Tang et al. 2012). A second mechanism involves modulation of primary regulatory structures and processes within the pontine brain stem. A study by Singleton et al. (2014) shed light on the possible mechanism of the much discussed impact of mindfulness practice on well-being; increases in well-being from mindfulness were correlated with increases in gray matter concentration in the dorsal pons. The correlation appears to support the mechanistic link between the well-being generated by mindfulness and the pontine nuclei of the mood- and arousal-modulating neurotransmitters serotonin, norepinephrine, and acetylcholine. This mechanism is supported by the findings of a study on the closely related practice of Zen meditation, which concluded that greater prefrontal activation and increased serotonin are correlated with improved mood in novice practitioners (Yu et al. 2011).

Although the study by Singleton et al. (2014) offers a plausible mechanism of how mindful mindset and mentality could support the affective component of self-transcendence, it is likely that the cognitive component involves alterations in the medullary brain stem, where the two vagal complexes intersect with the main centers of cardiorespiratory regulation and regenerative states. Early studies found that bare awareness practices linked with advanced breath control could elicit profoundly hypometabolic states akin to lucid hibernation (Heller et al. 1987), supporting paradoxically high levels of cortical arousal (Benson et al. 1982, 1990). More recent studies have replicated these findings (Amihai and Kozhevnikov 2014) and linked them to increased gray matter density in the medulla oblongata (Vestergaard-Poulsen et al. 2009). These related findings are consistent with Porges's (2011) theory that full integration of the brain stem social engagement system is supported by smart vagal modulation of primitive vagal freeze reactivity.

Conclusion: Mindfulness and the Future of Neuropsychiatry

In this chapter, I have brought together converging breakthroughs in neuroscience and physiology, including key elements of the emerging paradigm for psychiatry in the twenty-first century: allostasis, neural plasticity, social neuroscience, affective neuroscience, and polyvagal theory. The ways in which different forms of mindfulness help moderate traumatic stress reactivity and support social engagement at all levels of the nervous system further demonstrate the therapeutic benefits of mindful brain integration, rekindling the original promise of psychoanalysis to help bring unconscious structures and processes into the light of higher consciousness.

For clinicians, the single most remarkable and significant conclusion of this review is that mindfulness practices seem to share not only many of their beneficial effects but also their primary brain mechanisms with psychotherapy. This, in addition to the rising tide of neural research on these practices and the promising findings of mindfulness interventions in many conditions, makes a strong case for all mental health professionals to take an interest in the growing field of contemplative psychotherapy.

Key Points for Further Study and Reflection

- Basic mindfulness practice expands the size and capacity of the prefrontal and insular cortex, increasing self-awareness, attention, flexibility, interoception, and emotion regulation.
- Mindful sensitivity and loving-kindness practice expand the size of the anterior cingulate cortex and hippocampus, enhancing self-regulation of social emotions, responses, and rewards while reducing right amygdala size and bottom-up traumatic stress reactivity.
- Mindfulness of mindset and mentality promote the transcendence of aversive conditioning and default neuroendocrine and autonomic stress reactivity, by accessing and modulating subcortical and brain stem structures involved in implicit learning, internal reward, neuroendocrine rhythms, and autonomic tone.

- The five aspects of mindfulness practice overlap with other common contemplative practices, including Transcendental Meditation, the relaxation response, Hatha yoga, compassion training, Zen meditation, imagery, recitation, forced breathing, and mindful movement, providing an overview of the mechanisms and potential benefits of these practices for mental health and well-being.

References

Amihai I, Kozhevnikov M: Arousal vs. relaxation: a comparison of the neurophysiological and cognitive correlates of Vajrayana and Theravada meditative practices. PLoS One 9(7):e102990, 2014 25051268

Baer RA: Mindfulness training as a clinical intervention: a conceptual and empirical review. Clin Psychol Sci Pract 10:125–143, 2003

Beary JF, Benson H: A simple psychophysiologic technique which elicits the hypometabolic changes of the relaxation response. Psychosom Med 36(2):115–120, 1974 4814665

Benson H, Frankel FH, Apfel R, et al: Treatment of anxiety: a comparison of the usefulness of self-hypnosis and a meditational relaxation technique. An overview. Psychother Psychosom 30(3-4):229–242, 1978 368852

Benson H, Lehmann JW, Malhotra MS, et al: Body temperature changes during the practice of g Tum-mo yoga. Nature 295(5846):234–236, 1982 7035966

Benson H, Malhotra MS, Goldman RF, et al: Three case reports of the metabolic and electroencephalographic changes during advanced Buddhist meditation techniques. Behav Med 16(2):90–95, 1990 2194593

Brewer JA, Worhunsky PD, Gray JR, et al: Meditation experience is associated with differences in default mode network activity and connectivity. Proc Natl Acad Sci USA 108(50):20254–20259, 2011 22114193

Cahn BR, Polich J: Meditation states and traits: EEG, ERP, and neuroimaging studies. Psychol Bull 132(2):180–211, 2006 16536641

Creswell JD, Way BM, Eisenberger NI, Lieberman MD: Neural correlates of dispositional mindfulness during affect labeling. Psychosom Med 69(6):560–565, 2007 17634566

Dahl CJ, Lutz A, Davidson RJ: Reconstructing and deconstructing the self: cognitive mechanisms in meditation practice. Trends Cogn Sci 19(9):515–523, 2015 26231761

Davidson RJ: Affective style, psychopathology, and resilience: brain mechanisms and plasticity. Am Psychol 55(11):1196–1214, 2000 11280935

Davidson RJ: The Emotional Life of Your Brain. New York, Plume Books, 2013

Davidson RJ, Kabat-Zinn J, Schumacher J, et al: Alterations in brain and immune function produced by mindfulness meditation. Psychosom Med 65(4):564–570, 2003 12883106

DelMonte M: Meditation and the unconscious. J Contemp Psychother 25(3):223–242, 1995

Desbordes G, Negi LT, Pace TW, et al: Effects of mindful-attention and compassion meditation training on amygdala response to emotional stimuli in an ordinary, non-meditative state. Front Hum Neurosci 6:292, 2012 23125828

Epstein M: Thoughts Without a Thinker: Psychotherapy from a Buddhist Perspective. New York, NY, Basic Books, 1995

Farb NA, Segal ZV, Anderson AK: Mindfulness meditation training alters cortical representations of interoceptive attention. Soc Cogn Affect Neurosci 8(1):15–26, 2013 22689216

Fenwick PB: Meditation and the EEG, in The Psychology of Meditation. Edited by West MA. New York, Clarendon Press, 1987, pp 104–117

Fox KCR, Zakarauskas P, Dixon M, et al: Meditation experience predicts introspective accuracy. PLoS One 7(9):e45370, 2012 23049790

Fredrickson BL, Cohn MA, Coffey KA, et al: Open hearts build lives: positive emotions, induced through loving-kindness meditation, build consequential personal resources. J Pers Soc Psychol 95(5):1045–1062, 2008 18954193

Gard T, Taquet M, Dixit R, et al: Fluid intelligence and brain functional organization in aging yoga and meditation practitioners. Front Aging Neurosci 6:76, 2014 24795629

Gilbert P: The origins and nature of compassion focused therapy. Br J Clin Psychol 53(1):6–41, 2014 24588760

Goldin P, Ziv M, Jazaieri H, et al: MBSR vs aerobic exercise in social anxiety: fMRI of emotion regulation of negative self-beliefs. Soc Cogn Affect Neurosci 8(1):65–72, 2013 22586252

Goleman DJ, Schwartz GE: Meditation as an intervention in stress reactivity. J Consult Clin Psychol 44(3):456–466, 1976 777059

Gruzelier J: A theory of alpha/theta neurofeedback, creative performance enhancement, long distance functional connectivity and psychological integration. Cogn Process 10 (suppl 1):S101–S109, 2009 19082646

Harinath K, Malhotra AS, Pal K, et al: Effects of Hatha yoga and Omkar meditation on cardiorespiratory performance, psychologic profile, and melatonin secretion. J Altern Complement Med 10(2):261–268, 2004 15165407

Heller C, Elsner R, Rao N: Voluntary hypometabolism in an Indian Yogi. J Therm Biol 2:171–173, 1987

Hölzel BK, Carmody J, Evans KC, et al: Stress reduction correlates with structural changes in the amygdala. Soc Cogn Affect Neurosci 5(1):11–17, 2010 19776221

Hölzel BK, Carmody J, Vangel M, et al: Mindfulness practice leads to increases in regional brain gray matter density. Psychiatry Res 191(1):36–43, 2011a 21071182

Hölzel BK, Lazar SW, Gard T, et al: How does mindfulness meditation work? Proposing mechanisms of action from a conceptual and neural perspective. Perspect Psychol Sci 6(6):537–559, 2011b 26168376

Jang JH, Jung WH, Kang DH, et al: Increased default mode network connectivity associated with meditation. Neurosci Lett 487(3):358–362, 2011 21034792

Jha AP, Krompinger J, Baime MJ: Mindfulness training modifies subsystems of attention. Cogn Affect Behav Neurosci 7(2):109–119, 2007 17672382

Kabat-Zinn J: An outpatient program in behavioral medicine for chronic pain patients based on the practice of mindfulness meditation: theoretical considerations and preliminary results. Gen Hosp Psychiatry 4(1):33–47, 1982 7042457

Kandel ER: A new intellectual framework for psychiatry. Am J Psychiatry 155(4):457–469, 1998 9545989

Klimecki OM, Leiberg S, Lamm C, Singer T: Functional neural plasticity and associated changes in positive affect after compassion training. Cereb Cortex 23(7):1552–1561, 2013 22661409

Klimecki OM, Leiberg S, Ricard M, Singer T: Differential pattern of functional brain plasticity after compassion and empathy training. Soc Cogn Affect Neurosci 9(6):873–879, 2014 23576808

Kuyken W, Watkins E, Holden E, et al: How does mindfulness-based cognitive therapy work? Behav Res Ther 48(11):1105–1112, 2010 20810101

Lazar SW, Bush G, Gollub RL, et al: Functional brain mapping of the relaxation response and meditation. Neuroreport 11(7):1581–1585, 2000 10841380

Lazar SW, Kerr CE, Wasserman RH, et al: Meditation experience is associated with increased cortical thickness. Neuroreport 16(17):1893–1897, 2005 16272874

Leaviss J, Uttley L: Psychotherapeutic benefits of compassion-focused therapy: an early systematic review. Psychol Med 45(5):927–945, 2015 25215860

Linehan MM, Armstrong HE, Suarez A, et al: Cognitive-behavioral treatment of chronically parasuicidal borderline patients. Arch Gen Psychiatry 48(12):1060–1064, 1991 1845222

Loizzo J: Meditation and psychotherapy: stress, allostasis and enriched learning, in Complementary and Alternative Medicine and Psychiatry. Edited by Muskin PR. Review of Psychiatry, Vol 19 (Oldham JM, Riba MB, Series Editors). Washington, DC, American Psychiatric Press, 2000, pp 147–197

Loizzo J: Optimizing learning and quality of life throughout the lifespan: a global framework for research and application. Ann N Y Acad Sci 1172:186–198, 2009 19743554

Luders E, Toga AW, Lepore N, Gaser C: The underlying anatomical correlates of long-term meditation: larger hippocampal and frontal volumes of gray matter. Neuroimage 45(3):672–678, 2009 19280691

Luders E, Clark K, Narr KL, Toga AW: Enhanced brain connectivity in long-term meditation practitioners. Neuroimage 57(4):1308–1316, 2011 21664467

Luders E, Phillips OR, Clark K, et al: Bridging the hemispheres in meditation: thicker callosal regions and enhanced fractional anisotropy (FA) in long-term practitioners. Neuroimage 61(1):181–187, 2012 22374478

Luders E, Thompson PM, Kurth F, et al: Global and regional alterations of hippocampal anatomy in long-term meditation practitioners. Hum Brain Mapp 34(12):3369–3375, 2013 22815233

Lutz A, Greischar LL, Rawlings NB, et al: Long-term meditators self-induce high-amplitude gamma synchrony during mental practice. Proc Natl Acad Sci USA 101(46):16369–16373, 2004 15534199

Lutz A, Brefczynski-Lewis J, Johnstone T, Davidson RJ: Regulation of the neural circuitry of emotion by compassion meditation: effects of meditative expertise. PLoS One 3(3):e1897, 2008 18365029

MacLean KA, Ferrer E, Aichele SR, et al: Intensive meditation training improves perceptual discrimination and sustained attention. Psychol Sci 21(6):829–839, 2010 20483826

Mason LI, Alexander CN, Travis FT, et al: Electrophysiological correlates of higher states of consciousness during sleep in long-term practitioners of the Transcendental Meditation program. Sleep 20(2):102–110, 1997 9143069

Menon V: Large-scale brain networks and psychopathology: a unifying triple network model. Trends Cogn Sci 15(10):483–506, 2011 21908230

Neff KD: Self-compassion: an alternative conceptualization of a healthy attitude toward oneself. Self Ident 2:85–101, 2003

Pickut BA, Van Hecke W, Kerckhofs E, et al: Mindfulness based intervention in Parkinson's disease leads to structural brain changes on MRI: a randomized controlled longitudinal trial. Clin Neurol Neurosurg 115(12):2419–2425, 2013 24184066

Porges S: Polyvagal Theory: Neurophysiological Foundations of Emotions, Attachment, Communication and Self-Regulation. New York, WW Norton, 2011

Posner MI, Rothbart MK, Sheese BE, Tang Y: The anterior cingulate gyrus and the mechanism of self-regulation. Cogn Affect Behav Neurosci 7(4):391–395, 2007 18189012

Rosenzweig MR, Bennett EL: Psychobiology of plasticity: effects of training and experience on brain and behavior. Behav Brain Res 78(1):57–65, 1996 8793038

Rubin J: Psychotherapy and Buddhism: Toward an Integration. New York, Springer, 1996

Selye H: Stress and disease. Science 122:625–631, 1955

Shannahoff-Khalsa DS: Selective unilateral autonomic activation: implications for psychiatry. CNS Spectr 12(8):625–634, 2007 17667891

Siegel D: Pocket Guide to Interpersonal Neurobiology: An Integrative Handbook of the Mind. New York, WW Norton, 2012

Singleton O, Hölzel BK, Vangel M, et al: Change in brainstem gray matter concentration following a mindfulness-based intervention is correlated with improvement in psychological well-being. Front Hum Neurosci 18:8–33, 2014 24600370

Sperry R: Lateral specialization in the surgically separated hemispheres, in Third Neurosciences Study Program, Vol 3. Edited by Schmitt F, Worden F. Cambridge, MA, MIT Press, 1974, pp 5–19

Tang YY, Ma Y, Fan Y, et al: Central and autonomic nervous system interaction is altered by short-term meditation. Proc Natl Acad Sci USA 106(22):8865–8870, 2009 19451642

Tang YY, Rothbart MK, Posner MI: Neural correlates of establishing, maintaining, and switching brain states. Trends Cogn Sci 16(6):330–337, 2012 22613871

Teasdale JD, Segal Z, Williams JM: How does cognitive therapy prevent depressive relapse and why should attentional control (mindfulness) training help? Behav Res Ther 33(1):25–39, 1995 7872934

Telles S, Raghavendra BR, Naveen KV, et al: Changes in autonomic variables following two meditative states described in yoga texts. J Altern Complement Med 19(1):35–42, 2013 22946453

Vago D: Mapping modalities of self-awareness in mindfulness practice: a potential mechanism for clarifying habits of mind. Ann NY Acad Sci 1307:28–42, 2014 24117699

Vestergaard-Poulsen P, Van Beek M, Skewes J, et al: Long-term meditation is associated with increased gray matter density in the brain stem. Neuroreport 20(2):170–174, 2009 19104459

Weng HY, Fox AS, Shackman AJ, et al: Compassion training alters altruism and neural responses to suffering. Psychol Sci 24(7):1171–1180, 2013 23696200

Yu X, Fumoto M, Nakatani Y, et al: Activation of the anterior prefrontal cortex and serotonergic system is associated with improvements in mood and EEG changes induced by Zen meditation practice in novices. Int J Psychophysiol 80(2):103–111, 2011 21333699

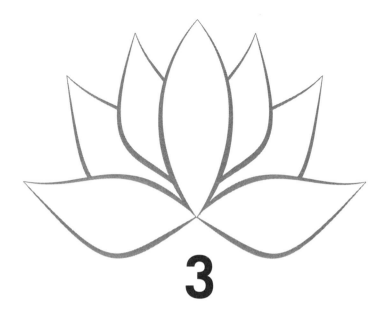

3

The Practice of Mindfulness

Kayleigh Pleas, MAPP
Cory Muscara, MAPP

Mindfulness is total clarity and presence of mind, actively passive, wherein events come and go like reflections in a mirror; nothing is reflected except what is.

Alan Watts, *The Way of Zen*

THE AMERICAN MONK Shinzen Young (2013) makes the helpful distinction between *mindfulness practices* and *mindfulness* itself. Mindful awareness practices are mind-training techniques designed to develop the following important attention skills:

- *Concentration power* gives us the capacity to focus and regulate our attention.
- *Sensory clarity* gives us the ability to notice the details of our sensory experience as it keeps changing.
- *Equanimity* gives us the ability to let our sensory experience come and go without resisting what is unpleasant or clinging onto what is pleasant.

These three skills enhance our capacity for mindful awareness itself, which, as discussed in Chapter 1, "What Is Mindfulness?," is simply moment-to-moment awareness of our present experience with curiosity, openness, and acceptance. Just as we can enhance base level physical fitness through specific, skillful training practices, so too can we enhance base level mindful awareness through specific, skillful mindful awareness practices.

In this chapter we explore three common mindfulness meditation practices that aim to cultivate the aforementioned skills:

- *Task-focused practice*, which aims to center the mind through focusing on a presently occurring phenomenon (i.e., the breath, bodily sensation, sound)
- *Open-monitoring practice*, which aims to cultivate a nonreactive orientation toward the ever-changing cascade of thoughts, sensations, and emotions occurring moment to moment
- *Loving-kindness and compassion meditation practice*, which aims to develop an attitude of care and tender-heartedness toward the self and others

Before we dive into these practices, we discuss the attitudinal qualities of mindfulness practice that distinguish this mindful awareness from basic perception, common misconceptions about the "goal" of mindfulness practice, formal versus informal practice, and helpful suggestions for starting a formal practice.[1]

---

[1] For you to effectively guide patients and clients in mindfulness practice, it is imperative that you develop a mindfulness practice of your own. The space that one inhabits in mindfulness meditation—nonjudgmental awareness—is a layer beneath the conceptual mind. Therefore, seeking to understand this practice through a conceptual lens can take you only so far. Mindfulness has to be experienced to be understood. Although this chapter serves as a map, the map is not the territory. In the same way that a mountaineer can guide others only through the external landscapes he or she has actually traveled, so too can a meditation teacher guide others only through the inner landscape of the human experience that he or she has traveled. The importance of this will be further outlined in Chapter 4, "Practice What You Preach."

Attitudinal Qualities of Mindfulness Practice

In their operational definition of *mindfulness*, Bishop et al. (2004) highlight two core aspects of the practice: 1) self-regulation of attention (concentration) and 2) an attitude that is curious and open (friendly). The gentle, accepting attitudinal stance is fundamental to mindfulness practice and cannot be overemphasized when working with a patient.

As we begin to see things clearly, such as emotional patterns of protection, physical discomfort, and painful truths, the embrace of friendliness allows us to hold whatever is arising without becoming critical or overwhelmed. In the same way that a therapist creates a safe space for his or her patient to investigate difficult thoughts, memories, and experiences, we as mindfulness practitioners need to create a safe space for ourselves to investigate difficult experiences. This gentle, accepting attitudinal perspective effectively creates a container in which we can navigate our own internal landscape.

Psychologist and meditation teacher Chris Germer (2009) likens this attitudinal stance to the way a mother gazes down at her newborn child: an embrace of unconditional love and acceptance. Germer states that "It's not possible to be aware of anything for very long if we're disgusted by it. We can experience the exquisite beauty of a rose, or a piece of music, or ourselves only if we are emotionally open" (Germer 2009, p. 42).

This attitudinal stance of friendliness could also be called compassionate awareness. Seeing things clearly (mindfulness) must be balanced with gentleness (compassion). As described by Bennett-Goleman (2001), the meditation teacher Tulku Urgyen Rinpoche described the relationship between mindfulness and compassion as two wings of a bird; without both wings, a bird cannot fly. As we begin to face the reality of our inner experience, compassion sustains us through periods that feel too difficult to bear. As mindfulness and compassion deepen, we discover an ever-present space of awareness within ourselves that can hold all of our feelings, discomforts, and reactions. Our relationship to everything that is arising and passing in our experience, pleasant and unpleasant, shifts as we rest more and more in awareness itself.

For a more comprehensive view of the attitudinal qualities of mindfulness, we turn to Jon Kabat-Zinn. In his first book, *Full Catastrophe Living*, Kabat-Zinn (1990) outlined seven attitudinal factors that are fundamental to the practice of mindfulness meditation. We offer a brief explanation of each of these attitudes, which should provide a framework for how one might view a moment of mindfulness. Additionally, these attitudinal factors serve as a reference for beginner students who are wondering if they are practicing "correctly."

1. *Nonjudging attitude*: We should try to take the perspective of an impartial witness to our own experience. As we begin to practice mindfulness, we quickly learn that our minds create judgments about nearly everything, particularly ourselves. It is important to simply recognize and observe these judgments without indulging in them.

2. *Patience*: We need to understand that sometimes things must unfold in their own time. There is often the tendency in mindfulness practice to speed up the process—that is, to try to become "peaceful" or "mindful" more quickly. The emergence of these qualities stems from a mind that is not trying to push past this current moment.

3. *Beginner's mind*: The great Zen meditation teacher Suzuki Roshi wrote, "In the beginner's mind there are many possibilities, but in the expert's there are few" (Suzuki 2010, p. 1). Over time, we develop a perceived expertise about ourselves, pigeonholing us into beliefs of what we can do and cannot do, who we are and who we are not. When we embrace this moment with curiosity and interest, as if we have never seen it before, there is infinite possibility for what it means and how we can respond to it. Additionally, much of the richness and beauty of our lives comes when we see something for the first time, like a child riding a slide. Maintaining a beginner's mind enables us to inhabit that space more often.

4. *Trust*: It is important that we develop a basic trust in ourselves and our feelings during meditation practice rather than override our intuition because we want to do it "right." If the meditation feels too emotionally charged to handle, we need to trust our instincts to step out of it for the time being and return when ready.

5. *Nonstriving attitude*: In our culture, we place great emphasis on achievement and getting things done. No doubt this has value, but to what end? If all we are doing is striving to get someplace else, then we are never actually living this moment of our lives. The effort and energy we exert in mindfulness practice is directed toward being present. The paradox is that in order to get anywhere, we need to stop striving to get there.

6. *Acceptance*: Acceptance is not passive resignation. It is the recognition that in this moment, things *are* the way things *are*. Until we can fully embrace our current reality, we cannot make informed decisions about what is best for us in this moment. Acceptance can often be painful because it means turning toward what we are most resisting or denying in our lives.

7. *Letting go*: Wanting control is a natural human tendency. When a good experience arises, we try to hold onto it, stretch it, and keep it for as long as possible; when a bad experience arises, we try to push it away, avoid it, and get rid of it as soon as possible. Each of these processes, pulling and pushing, creates some tension. Ultimately, these experiences come and go, no matter how much we want them to stay or not. In mindfulness, it is impor-

tant to practice observing these tendencies instead of incessantly reacting to them. There is a spaciousness and an ease that arises out of this.

Common Misperceptions: The *Goal* of Practice Versus the *By-Products* of Practice

With the ever-expanding scientific research celebrating the benefits of meditation, many people start a mindfulness practice with the goal of "fixing" what they don't like about themselves or their situation. Individuals new to meditation often hold the belief that "I can meditate away my stress" or "If I get good enough at meditating, then all my problems will go away."

Although individuals who practice mindfulness regularly often experience less anxiety in daily life, enhanced mood, and improved health, these are by-products of mindfulness, not the goal. The goal of mindfulness is to cultivate greater awareness and acceptance of what is happening, right here, in the present moment. This process of not trying to get someplace better is counterintuitive to our cultural strategy of personal development. However, when we approach ourselves with this type of curiosity and gentleness (tenderhearted acceptance) and have no expectation of getting something or fixing what we don't like, our relationship to our experience shifts simply by paying attention. Observing the arising and passing of an emotion, physical sensation, thought, or mental image—bringing precise awareness to the component parts of the experience—loosens our identification with it. Instead of being consumed by the thought, feeling, or sensation and reacting to it, we are free to respond to the ever-changing flow of our human experience from the abiding awareness that is noticing. Here, freedom from the habitual reactions that limit our self-understanding and potential for happiness is possible.

Mindfulness offers a radical shift in how we relate to the stress and pain in our lives and, more broadly, how we understand and approach the entirety of our human experience. Instead of trying to get somewhere, achieve a goal, or fix something, we learn to be present, open, and accepting of what is.

Formal Versus Informal Practice

Formal practice refers to the period of time we carve out of our day to do a structured mindful awareness practice (e.g., focusing on the sensation of breath, scanning the body, repeating loving-kindness phrases). Although the aim of this chapter is to offer instruction in the practice of formal mindful awareness practices, informal practice is equally important.

Informal practice refers to bringing mindful awareness to our daily activities and engagements by noticing bodily sensations, thoughts, emotions, and surroundings as we move through the tasks of daily life. Any time we bring our attention to the present moment with an attitude of curiosity, openness, and gentleness, we are practicing mindfulness. Thus, we can practice mindfulness at any moment—while walking, eating, listening, washing the dishes, or hugging. Simply bringing our full attention to what we are doing and experiencing in the present moment is the ultimate aim of mindfulness.

Many people find informal practice more approachable than formal practice, especially when they are new to mindfulness. We do not need to "do" anything special; we just need to pay attention in a different way. For example, when taking a shower, instead of being lost in thoughts about the day or concerns about yesterday, we can choose to be present to the experience of showering: feel the sensation of water on our skin, the tub or shower beneath our feet, the breath in our belly. We choose to bring our attention back to the experience of showering when we notice our mind wanders off. *This* is mindfulness.

Informal practice is particularly helpful when we feel stressed, anxious, depressed, or angry. Stopping in a moment of emotional overwhelm to notice what is happening with curiosity and tenderness interrupts the habits of reaction that cause the greatest suffering, providing the space to observe our experience rather than react to it. Some helpful questions to ask in a moment of overwhelm include these: What is happening in my body? (Contraction in my chest? Tingling in my fingers? Fluttering in my stomach?) What emotions are present? (Fear? Confusion? Anger? Sorrow?) What is happening in my mind with my thinking? (Thoughts about the future? The past? Myself? Others?) Pausing in a moment of overwhelm to "be with" what is happening requires stopping and observing ourselves and our situation with curiosity and interest, not judging or trying to fix it but just noticing and turning toward it. One mindful pause is enough to give ourselves the inner resources to respond, rather than to react, to whatever is happening around us.

One might read this and think, "Well, I'm just going to do informal practice all the time; that sounds much easier." However, an important relationship here is that our formal practice informs and supports our informal practice. For us to be able to tap into informal practice in a skillful and meaningful way, we must simultaneously be exercising this capacity during formal meditation sessions.

Helpful Suggestions for Starting a Formal Practice

Meditation Posture

Although you can practice attention and awareness in any bodily posture (standing on your head or hunching over your computer), the posture you assume does facilitate levels of energy and comfort in the body, particularly during extended meditation periods.

To start, find a seated posture that allows you to sit upright but not uptight, resting as easefully as possible in a chair with your feet rooted on the floor or on a cushion with legs crossed. Balance your head over your shoulders and shoulders over your hips and keep your spine straight and relaxed. Use as little effort as possible to hold yourself up. You may rest your hands on your thighs, palms down or up, or cup one hand in the other in your lap. Draw your chin back slightly toward your chest to lengthen the back of the neck. Close your eyes, or if it is more comfortable for you, rest your eyes on an object about 3 feet in front of you and soften your gaze.

Settling In

Take a moment to welcome yourself into your physical body and feel yourself present. Offer a curious and gentle attention to your hands, feet, face, shoulders, chest, belly, and legs. Notice any areas that may be holding unnecessary tension—typically around the eyes and jaw, between the shoulders, deep in the belly or hips—and invite them to soften.

Call to mind your intention in choosing to practice. Intentions may include alleviating suffering, loving more fully, experiencing freedom from fear, or knowing joy. Grounding the mind in a positive intention helps stabilize your attention and motivates wise effort and commitment.

Using a Timer

Many people, especially beginners, find setting a timer for formal practice extremely helpful. No matter where your mind wanders or what arises, the time you set aside is safeguarded for you. Simply invite your attention back until the timer rings. Beginning with 5 minutes is often sustainable for people. As this becomes a comfortable habit, you may increase your time to 10 minutes and expand from there.

The Three Primary Mindful Awareness Practices

Task-Focused Practice

Task-focused practice involves focusing our attention, like a flashlight, on a specific, presently occurring event—such as a sound, bodily sensation, breath, or physical touch—that serves as an *anchor* for the mind. Naturally, as we direct our attention toward our object of focus, a host of thoughts, feelings, bodily sensations, and distractions arise. When we notice that we have left the present—

meandering off into planning, resisting, judging, or dreaming—the task is to kindly invite ourselves back to our anchor.

Our greatest suffering arises from a mind lost in thought—ruminating about the past, worrying about the future, or being preoccupied by a difficult emotion. A sensory anchor gives the mind a neutral stimulus to return to, allowing us to re-establish the steadiness needed to navigate our ever-changing human experience.

An attitude of kindness is important. We want to relate to ourselves the way a supportive parent attends to a child, tenderly and directly. Many of us are so accustomed to being harsh with ourselves that we bring the same harshness into our meditation practice. Use an inner tone that is warm and friendly, even play-ful. An excellent piece of advice that one of us received early in practice was to notice when the mind wanders off into thinking and then to smile and say to yourself, "I see you, monkey mind!"

Common Task-Focused Practices

The lists below outline three common task-focused practices that can be used to cul-tivate mindfulness. As you navigate each of these practices, incorporate the attitu-dinal qualities of mindfulness that we have been discussing throughout this chapter.

Mindfulness of Sound

- Set a timer for anywhere between 3 and 10 minutes.
- Sit in an upright, relaxed position, spine straight and comfortable, with your eyes closed.
- Gently scan through your body, inviting any areas holding tension to soften.
- Set the intention to notice sound. You can say to yourself, "Now, I choose to listen to sound." Sound is the anchor for your attention.
- Allow sounds to come to you, noticing how the vibration of sound occurs and passes away. You do not need to search for sounds or push sounds away; simply allow one sound to come and then the next.
- When you notice that your mind wanders away from sound, invite yourself back to listen.
- Your mind will automatically start to label sounds, judge sounds as pleasant or unpleasant, and wander into distraction. Expect this to happen. When you notice you have left sound, kindly and firmly invite yourself back.
- Be with the symphony of sounds as they change, neither liking nor disliking.
- When your timer chimes, congratulate yourself for taking the time to practice.

Mindfulness of the Breath

- Set a timer for anywhere between 3 and 10 minutes.
- Sit in an upright, relaxed position, spine straight and comfortable, with eyes closed.

- Gently scan through your body, inviting any areas holding tension to soften.
- Set the intention to notice your breath. You can say to yourself, "Now, I choose to observe my breath." The breath is the anchor for your attention.
- Begin by noticing the many sensations and movements that are present during an inhalation and exhalation. You may observe the expanding and contracting of the chest, the rising and falling of the shoulders, or movement in the belly.
- Eventually, anchor your attention to one particular aspect of the breath. We recommend focusing on the belly (i.e., the rising and falling of the abdomen) because doing so often facilitates a deeper breathing.
- When you notice that your mind wanders away from the breath, gently invite yourself back to this moment of breathing.
- If you would like, you may count in your head after each breath, making a note of 1, then 2, and so on, up to 10. If you lose your place, start over with 1. Even if you just count to 3 over and over again, what is most important is that you recognize that your mind has wandered and then bring it back again. This recognition that your mind has wandered and then returning to the task is as much a part of the meditation as the sustained attention on the task itself. The numbers simply serve to help you notice when your attention has wandered.
- When your timer chimes, congratulate yourself for taking the time to practice.

Note about using the breath as your anchor: People who have experienced physical trauma may feel uncomfortable bringing awareness into the body through the breath. People with physical health anxieties or body shame may also find meditating on the breath too overwhelming. Compulsive, controlling types of people may find that focusing on the breath creates restriction and a gripping in the breath. If any of these situations should occur, use a different anchor for the practice—the feeling of one's feet on the floor or an object outside the body such as the sensation of holding a stone or gazing at a flower.

Mindfulness of the Body

- Set a timer for anywhere between 3 and 10 minutes.
- Sit in an upright, relaxed position, spine straight and comfortable, with eyes closed. (If you are able to lie on the floor, that is another option for this practice.)
- Gently scan through your body, inviting any areas holding tension to soften.
- Rest your attention on your breath for a few moments to settle in and ground yourself.
- Begin by noticing the sensations in your feet with a nonjudgmental awareness. If you do not notice any sensations, be aware of the experience of *non*-sensation.

- Continue navigating your awareness up your body, moving from the feet to the shins/calves, knees, thighs, pelvis, back, belly, chest, arms/hands, shoulders, neck, face, and top of head.
- The tendency is to sometimes visualize the body part. Notice when this happens and instead tune into the sensations, or the *felt* experience, of this body part.
- When you notice that your mind wanders away from whatever part of your body you are focusing on, gently invite yourself back to it.
- If any particular region of the body feels too uncomfortable or overwhelming to focus on, experiment with navigating the outer edges of that region. For instance, if the pelvis is a sensitive area, notice what it is like to observe the sensations of the thigh right where it begins integrating with the sensations of the pelvis. The thigh is your "safe" zone that you can go back to in this scenario.
- At the end of the body scan, feel your body as a whole, sitting or lying there in space.
- When your timer chimes, congratulate yourself for taking the time to practice.

Note about using the body as your anchor: Most people have some form of self-consciousness about their bodies, ranging from minor to extreme. When you introduce this practice to people, it is very important to emphasize the attitudinal quality of nonjudgment. Also, for patients with trauma, this can be a very intense practice; if you know someone has a traumatic history, have the individual start this practice with eyes open and let the person know that he or she can stop at any point.

Practice Tips: Noting and Labeling

A helpful method for sustaining attention is to use noting and labeling.

- *Noting* is the process of turning toward an inner experience (thought, feeling, or sensation) as it arises to make a mental note. Without going deeply into the experience, acknowledge the experience ("Oh, this") and return to your anchor.
- *Labeling* is the process of giving a specific title to an inner experience. For instance, when you notice a thought come through your mind, you might label it "thinking." If you notice boredom arise, label it "boredom." If anger arises, label it "anger." By doing this practice you are seeing and identifying an experience for exactly what it is, without an extra "story" or mental narrative about the experience.

Benefits and By-Products of Task-Focused Practice

- Calms the mind-body
- Anchors mind in the present

- Reverses the tendency to avoid or resist emotional pain
- Balances awareness of pain
- Provides stability of mind that allows you to examine your experience

Challenges Experienced Early in Task-Focused Practice

- *"I don't have the mind for meditation. I can't do it."* Early in meditation practice, one quickly learns how busy and distracted one's mind is. Half a breath in, and you may be off planning tomorrow, ruminating about yesterday, or lost in fantasy. One of the most common misunderstandings is believing that you "can't meditate" because your mind is so distracted. The mind is actually designed to wander, looking for novelty and stimulation. Distractions are part of the meditation process. Every time you notice your mind has wandered, you are having a moment of mindfulness. The hallmark of an advanced practitioner is not a perfectly still mind but rather the willingness to return to the breath, again and again, without judgment.
- *"Meditating increases my anxiety."* Many people come to meditation with the expectation that they should feel relaxed and calm. Try approaching meditation without any expectation for what should or should not happen. When you sit with yourself for more than a few minutes, all the feelings you have not wanted to acknowledge, physical discomforts, and fears will eventually arise. The mind will always find something to dredge up. The goal of meditation is not to improve yourself or fix something you do not like. The goal of meditation is to be with whatever is happening with curiosity and gentleness, providing insight into *how the mind works*.

Open-Monitoring Practice

Open-monitoring practice entails observing the constant fluctuation of internal bodily sensations, thoughts, and emotions without attaching to them or pushing them away. A helpful analogy is to imagine awareness itself as a spacious, luminous sky. As weather systems move across the sky, the sky remains unaffected, neither clinging onto a passing cloud nor pushing it away.

The purpose of practice is not to change our experience but to change our reaction to our experience. Over time, we learn to perceive and relate to our emotional states with clarity, curiosity, and acceptance. The brains of advanced meditators show diminished activity in stress-related areas of the brain.

Choiceless Awareness

- Set a timer for anywhere between 3 and 10 minutes.
- Sit in an upright, relaxed position, spine straight and comfortable, with eyes closed. (If you are able to lie on the floor, that is another option for this practice.)

- Gently scan through your body, inviting any areas holding tension to soften.
- Rest your attention on your breath for a few moments to settle in and ground yourself.
- Once you feel settled, you can allow your attention to move away from the breath, so that you are not attending to any "thing" in particular. Instead, you are just resting in awareness, noticing whatever arises in your experience.
- Don't hold on to anything, look for anything, or try to create any experience. Simply be receptive to and aware of whatever comes in and out of your experience, similar to what happens as you look out the window of your car as trees, animals, signs, and the sky pass by.
- When your timer chimes, congratulate yourself for taking the time to practice.

A Moment of Mindful Presence

You can establish a mindful presence any time you stop to recognize what is going on in and around yourself. Helpful questions: What sensations are present in my body? How am I feeling? What am I thinking about? What is going on around me?

When you find yourself stressed and overwhelmed, consider the acronym STOP as a reminder of how to reengage with mindful presence:

- Stop.
- Take a breath.
- Observe nonjudgmentally what you are experiencing in your mind and body.
- Proceed with awareness and grounding.

Challenges to Open-Monitoring Practice

- Open-monitoring practice can be difficult for beginners, especially after practicing task-focused meditation. Without a particular anchor (sounds, breath, body) on which to direct your attention, you might start wondering, "What should I be focusing on?" A helpful question to ask yourself is, "What is here now?" You may discover a feeling of doubt about whether or not you are doing the practice correctly or frustration that this practice feels more difficult. In open-monitoring practice, these mind states and emotions, whatever is here *now*, become your object of awareness.
- With this said, the practice can still be overwhelming in the beginning, even with the aforementioned instructions. Therefore, if it becomes too difficult or frustrating, you can always return to an anchor with which you feel comfortable and grounded—sounds, breath, or body—and once you feel settled again, you can practice letting go of that anchor, simply resting in awareness of whatever arises.

Benefits and By-Products of Open-Monitoring Practice

- Insight into the nature of how the mind works (the longer you spend in meditation, the more you learn about the inner workings of the mind and the tendency of the mind to wander off into judgment, comparison, and worry)
- Enhanced creativity
- Feelings of spaciousness; fewer restrictions
- Practical application into daily life; simply noticing what is going on around you
- Expansive view of yourself (bigger than your thoughts, emotions, or pain)

Loving-Kindness and Compassion Meditation Practice: Cultivating the Heart

Loving-kindness and compassion meditation practice is designed to actualize our potential for tenderhearted connection with ourselves and all beings. Whereas task-focused practices help steady the mind and open-monitoring practices help us meet our ever-changing experience with calm balance, loving-kindness and compassion practices help us turn toward the vulnerability of being alive with an all-embracing, immeasurable love. The Buddha described the path of practice as "the liberation of the heart which is love" (Salzberg 2002, p. 1).

Although loving-kindness and compassion are similar in tone, they are different. *Loving-kindness* is the wish for another person, or oneself, to experience happiness. *Mettā*, the Pali word for loving-kindness, can also be translated as "unconditional friendliness" or benevolence. We can experience loving-kindness any time we cultivate an attitude of goodwill toward another or ourselves.

Compassion, on the other hand, is the wish for another person, or oneself, to be free from suffering. Meditation teacher Sharon Salzberg (2002) describes compassion as the "strength that arises out of seeing the true nature of suffering in the world. Compassion allows us to bear witness to that suffering, whether it is in ourselves or others, without fear; it allows us to name injustice without hesitation, and to act strongly" (Salzberg 2002, p. 103). Compassion occurs when we notice suffering and feel motivated to alleviate that suffering through an inner wish or external action. For practical purposes, compassion meditation can be thought of as a subset of loving-kindness meditation (Germer 2009).

Loving-Kindness Practice

Loving-kindness meditation is a form of single-focus meditation that uses phrases, as opposed to the breath, as the anchor of attention. The purpose of the practice is to connect with our shared human desire for happiness by cultivating an attitude of good will first toward the self and then to an ever-expanding circle of others. Common *Mettā* phrases used in the practice include these: *May I be safe. May I be happy. May I be healthy. May I live with ease.*

Traditionally, there are six categories of people toward whom we gradually open our hearts in loving-kindness: 1) self—our own precious human life; 2) benefactor—someone who brightens our heart and makes us smile, like a mentor, spiritual guide, or child; 3) friend—someone we care for, respect, and feel supported by; 4) neutral person—someone we don't know and neither like nor dislike; 5) difficult person—someone we don't like because he or she has caused us pain; and 6) groups—large clusters of people, like the people in our workplace, city, state, or country.

Note: Move through the six categories at your own pace and in an order that feels natural. Because so many of us struggle with self-judgment and self-loathing, starting with the benefactor is a skillful way of warming up our hearts enough to eventually make space for ourselves in loving-kindness. The difficult person category will give rise to a host of emotions and should be practiced only when you feel ready.

- Set a timer for 10–20 minutes.
- Sit in an upright, relaxed, comfortable position.
- Close your eyes and bring your attention to the sensations around your heart.
- Reflect on your intention to awaken your capacity for love and tenderheartedness.
- Connect with your most sincere wish for happiness and peace, and remember that this wish connects you to every living being on the planet.
- Turn toward the life that is right here in your body the way you would turn toward a good friend. Think something like, "Just as all beings wish to be happy and free from suffering, may I be happy and free from suffering." Try to feel the warmth of your loving intention in your body, softening your chest, shoulders, face, and hands.
- Repeat the following *Mettā* phrases silently with a warm inner tone of voice: *May I be safe. May I be happy. May I be healthy. May I live with ease.*
- Absorb the meaning of each phrase, allowing the words to sift down into you.
- Go slowly. Savor the intention behind each word.
- When your mind wanders away from your phrases, simply notice that you have wandered and invite yourself back to your phrases.
- After spending some time offering loving-kindness to yourself, call to mind someone who naturally makes you smile, such as a mentor, spiritual figure, or child. Visualize this person and let your heart be touched by his or her goodness and shared wish for happiness. Direct the *Mettā* phrases toward your benefactor, surrounding him or her in loving-kindness: *May you be safe. May you be happy. May you be healthy. May you live with ease.*

- Now call to mind a friend, someone you know well, care for, and feel supported by. Visualize this person and let your heart be touched by his or her goodness and shared wish for happiness. Direct the *Mettā* phrases toward your friend, surrounding him or her in loving-kindness: *May you be safe. May you be happy. May you be healthy. May you live with ease.*
- Next, call to mind a neutral person, someone whose face you can imagine, but whose story you don't know (e.g., your local grocery clerk, a neighbor you pass on the street, a colleague at work). Let your heart be touched by this other's humanity and your shared desire to lead a life of happiness. Direct the same phrases toward this neutral person.
- Call to mind a difficult person in your life. It is best to start with someone who is only mildly difficult, not someone associated with a traumatic experience. Remember that people who cause suffering to others are themselves suffering. Gently repeat the *Mettā* phrases while keeping an image of this person in your mind. It is natural that feelings of anger, disgust, aversion, or sadness arise. Label the emotion as it arises without judgment ("Oh, anger"), and offer yourself loving-kindness if you need to. When you feel ready, return to the image of the difficult person.
- Continue to offer your wish of loving-kindness toward an ever-expanding circle of others—friends and family and people you know only remotely. Allow their names and/or faces to arise in your mind, and as each arises, offer the same intention of loving-kindness by repeating the phrases.
- Eventually, expand your feelings of love and kindness to all people and creatures on the planet. You may do this by visualizing groupings of people—people in your city, your region, your continent, and finally the whole world.
- Imagine the billions of human beings doing their best to make meaning of their lives, who, like you, want to experience peace and happiness. Continue to repeat the phrases, gently and kindly: *May all beings be safe. May all beings be happy. May all beings be healthy. May all beings live with ease.*
- When your timer chimes, let go of the phrases and spend a few moments resting in the power of your intention.
- Notice what is happening in your body with kind curiosity.
- Whatever you experienced or did not experience, rest in the power of your intention to offer unconditional friendliness to yourself and all beings.

Compassion Meditation Practice

Compassion meditation is a form of single-focus meditation that uses phrases as the anchor of attention. The purpose of the practice is to transform our relationship to suffering, whether it is our own or that of another. Suffering is an intrinsic part of life that we cannot avoid. Through the practice, we learn to acknowledge suffering, open to it, and respond with courage and kindness. This allows us to "hold" difficulty—our own or another's—without getting overwhelmed or feeling isolated. Traditionally, only one or two phrases, perhaps phrases like these, are used: *May you be free from inner and outer harm. May you know peace.* Tailor the phrases so they are meaningful to you.

- Set a timer for 10–20 minutes.
- Sit in an upright, relaxed, comfortable position.
- Close your eyes and bring your attention to the sensations around your heart.
- Reflect on your intention to awaken your capacity for compassion. Connect with your most sincere wish for the alleviation of suffering, your own and the suffering of all.
- Bring to mind someone with great physical or mental suffering. Without taking on this person's story, let your heart be touched by his or her situation. Envelop this person in compassion by silently repeating these phrases (or phrases of your choice): *May you be free from inner and outer harm. May you know peace.*
- Now turn toward the life that is right here in your heart, mind, and body— your precious human life. Notice any physical or mental suffering present in you, and let your heart be touched by your own experience.
- Envelop yourself with compassion by silently repeating these phrases (or phrases of your choice): *May I be free from inner and outer harm. May I know peace.*
- Continue to expand your offering of compassion toward an ever-expanding circle of others: benefactor, good friend, neutral person, difficult person, all your friends and family, all people and beings across the globe.
- Go at your own pace, moving from person to person as you feel inclined. Allow the meaning of the words to be experienced.
- When your timer chimes, let go of the phrases and rest in the power of your intention.
- Notice what is happening in your body with kind curiosity.
- Whatever you experienced or did not experience, rest in the power of your intention to offer compassion to yourself and all beings.

Helpful Tips for Loving-Kindness and Compassion Meditation Practice

- Develop your own phrases. Any phrases that feel authentic and inspiring to you are appropriate. Examples include these: *May you accept yourself as you are. May you feel loved. May you be kind to yourself. May you care for yourself with ease.* Once you decide on your phrases, stick with them.

- Use imagery. Many people find imagery to be a powerful way to engage the feelings of loving-kindness and compassion. Imagine your loved one very close up. See him or her receive your wish for happiness.
- Use an inner tone that reflects your tenderhearted intention. Repeat the phrases to yourself the way you would speak to a good friend.

Challenges to Loving-Kindness and Compassion Practice

- *"I feel cold or numb."* We often don't feel warm and tender when practicing, and that is OK. Forming an intention in our mind for happiness is different from trying to strong-arm our inner experience and force certain feelings. As Salzberg (2002) says, we are simply "planting seeds by forming this powerful intention in the mind" and settling back, curious and open to observe without judgment (p. 39).
- *"I don't think I deserve loving-kindness."* Offering ourselves kindness is often confused with being self-indulgent or self-centered. The first step toward loving others is loving ourselves. We are better able to serve others when we ourselves are happy and free from suffering.
- *"I feel overwhelming guilt, shame, or worthlessness when I practice."* Loving-kindness practice will inevitably bring up any unexamined emotional pain. Germer (2009) refers to this process as "back draft" (p. 150). In the same way that a smoldering fire deprived of oxygen will erupt into greater flames when met with air, so too any smoldering feelings of self-judgment or self-hatred will erupt when met with loving awareness. Expect difficult feelings to arise. Don't try to push them away or fight them by intensifying loving-kindness; rather, apply mindfulness. Notice what is arising without judgment. If you feel overwhelmed, turn to your breath as an anchor, letting go of the phrases until you feel ready to resume.
- *"The phrases have become meaningless or hollow."* In any meditation using words as the focus of the meditation, the words will eventually lose their potency. When this happens, remind yourself why you are practicing by reflecting on your intention.
- *"I feel fear, despair, sorrow, or anger."* Accept that this is a normal part of the practice. Notice without judgment what you are feeling and bring your attention to your breath. Anchor your awareness in your breath until you feel ready to begin again. If an emotion is overwhelming, you may try labeling the emotion in a supportive voice ("Oh, this is sadness") or locating the emotion in your body (e.g., chest, belly, throat) as the sensations keep changing.

Benefits and By-Products of Loving-Kindness and Compassion Practice

- Developing the equanimity needed to turn toward difficult emotions, rather than numbing or over-identifying with them
- Ability to feel warmth toward someone, including yourself, who is suffering
- Acceptance and compassion toward others and yourself
- Feelings of social connection and positive relationships with others
- Increases in daily experiences of positive emotion, including love, gratitude, hope, awe, and amusement
- Improved mindful awareness in everyday life
- Greater life satisfaction
- Improved physical health

Key Points for Further Study and Reflection

- Just as an individual can enhance base level physical fitness through specific, skillful training practices, so too can an individual enhance base level mindful awareness through specific, skillful mindful awareness practices.
- Three common mindfulness meditation practices include *task-focused practice*, which aims to center the mind through focusing on a presently occurring phenomenon (i.e., sound, the breath, bodily sensation); *open-monitoring practice*, which aims to cultivate a nonreactive orientation toward the ever-changing cascade of thoughts, sensations, and emotions occurring moment to moment; and *compassion and loving-kindness practices*, which aim to develop an attitude of care and tender-heartedness toward self and others.
- Through daily practice, we discover a space of awareness within ourselves that allows us to respond, rather than react, to our ever-changing human experience with wisdom and compassion.

References

Bennett-Goleman T: Emotional Alchemy: How the Mind Can Heal the Heart. New York, Three Rivers Press, 2001

Bishop SR, Lau M, Shapiro S, et al: Mindfulness: a proposed operational definition. Clin Psychol Sci Pract 11(3):230–241, 2004

Germer CK: The Mindful Path to Self-Compassion: Freeing Yourself From Destructive Thoughts and Emotions. New York, Guilford, 2009

Kabat-Zinn J: Full Catastrophe Living: Using the Wisdom of Your Body and Mind to Face Stress, Pain, and Illness. New York, Delacorte, 1990

Salzberg S: Lovingkindness: The Revolutionary Art of Happiness. Boston, MA, Shambhala, 2002

Suzuki S: Zen Mind, Beginner's Mind. Boston, MA, Shambhala, 2010

Young S: What Is Mindfulness? 2013. Available at: http://www.shinzen.org/Articles/WhatIsMindfulness_SY_Public.pdf. Accessed February 1, 2016.

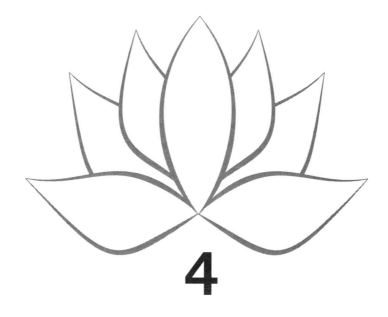

4

Practice What You Preach

The Mindful Clinician

Rebecca Hedrick, M.D.
Andrea Brandon, M.D.
Seema Desai, M.D.

When practicing mindfully, clinicians approach their everyday tasks with critical curiosity. They are present in the moment, seemingly undistracted, able to listen before expressing an opinion, and able to be calm even if they are doing several things at once. These qualities are considered by many to be a prerequisite for compassionate care.

Ronald M. Epstein (2003)

CLINICIANS TYPICALLY think of mindfulness as a tool they can teach patients, yet research findings suggest that becoming a mindful clinician has many additional benefits. Mindfulness can help to cultivate an attitude of compassion, increase empathy for patients, improve a clinician's ability to attend to patients in sessions, and decrease clinician burnout (Irving et al. 2009). Thus, patients benefit from clinician mindfulness regardless of whether mindfulness instruction is provided to the patient.

When we as clinicians do intend to explicitly bring mindfulness practices into our patient sessions, it is vital that we embody the qualities of mindfulness by having a committed personal practice. To navigate the terrain of the mind, we must have a good understanding of the map. Without our own mindfulness practice, it is challenging to guide patients using mindfulness principles. In this chapter we focus on clinician mindfulness, exploring the benefits to both the clinician and the patient; techniques to cultivate clinician mindfulness; and universal barriers and obstacles to a mindfulness practice, as well as hindrances that are more specific to clinicians.

Benefits of Mindfulness for the Clinician

Cultivation of Attitudes and Therapeutic Presence

Clinician mindfulness training has been shown to improve the effectiveness of healers by cultivating many qualities, including the following (Davis and Hayes 2011; Germer et al. 2013; Irving et al. 2009):

- Enhanced attention—purposeful and sustained focus of awareness on selected experience
- Emotional intelligence—ability to recognize, differentiate, and regulate emotions within oneself and others and to use emotional information to guide and inform thoughts and behavior
- Social connectedness—ability to relate to others and one's self with kindness, acceptance, and compassion (Davis and Hayes 2011)

- Empathy—emotional attunement to the patient's experience that helps the patient to feel understood
- Compassion—attunement to the patient's suffering, accompanied by the desire to alleviate it
- Affect tolerance—ability to remain present, without becoming overwhelmed or flooded, when patients express intense, difficult emotions
- Equanimity—emotional imperturbability along with a radical acceptance of things as they are without attachment to results

By strengthening these personal and interpersonal qualities, mindfulness allows the clinician to bring more of his or her caring "self" to the patient interaction. These qualities also generate a therapeutic presence, defined as "an availability and openness to all aspects of the [patient's] experience, openness to one's own experience in being with the [patient], and the capacity to respond to the [patient] from this experience" (McCollum and Gehart 2010, p. 347). This presence promotes a discerning but noncondemning critical curiosity that does not box a patient into a narrow diagnosis or treatment but can honor the complexity of the individual as a whole. In these ways, clinician mindfulness may lead to improved clinical judgment, decreased patient errors, more effective healing, and improvements in quality of care and patient outcomes (Epstein 2003).

Reduction of Burnout

The high prevalence of clinician burnout in the fields of medicine and mental health has been the subject of many recent publications. In a profession that attracts and rewards self-sacrifice for the good of others without placing much of a premium on self-care, burnout is an occupational hazard. Emotional exhaustion, cynicism toward work, and reduced sense of personal accomplishment characterize burnout, which in some studies has been reported in up to 60% of practicing clinicians (Krasner et al. 2009). Clinician burnout has been linked to impaired patient care and to serious health consequences for the clinician (Irving et al. 2009; Shapiro and Carlson 2009, p. 117).

Mindfulness cultivates healthy mental, emotional, and physical changes and is therefore ideally suited to prevent and treat the multifaceted and complex cycle of burnout. Mindfulness facilitates the self-awareness that can enable the clinician to notice the early signs of burnout, including feelings of dread about going to work, excessive boredom, feelings of flatness or tiredness, and pessimism about the future. Moreover, working with mindfulness promotes compassion and equanimity, which further serve to mitigate burnout. Results of research suggest that clinician participation in mindfulness programs can minimize burnout by decreasing rates of anxiety, stress, and depression, as well as increasing self-compassion, gratitude, relaxation, life satisfaction, and positive affect (Davis and Hayes 2011; Irving et al. 2009).

Establishing a Mindfulness Practice for the Clinician

Formal Practice for the Clinician

Clinician mindfulness can be cultivated through formal and informal practices. Formal practice—what is normally called meditation—is an "opportunity to experience mindfulness at its deepest levels. Sustained, disciplined introspection allows the practitioner to train attention, systematically observe the mind's contents, and learn how the mind works" (Germer et al. 2013, p. 15). A clinician can engage in formal practice through daily meditation, joining a training program or a meditation group, attending a designated meditation retreat, and working with a teacher.

Establish a Daily Practice

There are many ways in which you can practice mindfulness. The goal is to develop a regular practice that helps you to train your mind. No matter what practice you choose, from mindful movement to seated meditation, it will take commitment, patience, and gentle discipline. The following tips have been adapted from Kornfield (1993, p. 65).

Tips to Establish a Daily Mindfulness Practice

- Commit to a regular time of day for practice.
- Begin with a few minutes a day and gradually work your way up to longer times.
- Find a quiet location where you can remain undisturbed.
- Choose a type of meditation that resonates with you and stick with it.
- Be kind to yourself.
- There is no right or wrong way—just practice.

Try a Training Program

Enrolling in a Mindfulness-Based Stress Reduction or Mindfulness-Based Cognitive Therapy training program is one way to jump-start your own practice. Programs usually last 8–12 weeks and teach various skills, including mindful breathing, mindful walking, mindful eating, and formal sitting meditation. Not only will you learn skills to teach patients but you will acquire those skills yourself and find a group of people with whom to practice. These programs often offer the opportunity to engage in ongoing group practice after the course is completed.

Find a Teacher

Having a good teacher and mentor is generally an integral component of developing a mindfulness practice. A teacher can help you learn faster and keep you on track from potential pitfalls associated with practice. Finding a teacher is an individual journey, but some general guidelines are useful: The search for a teacher may begin with recommendations from trusted persons or Web sites or from articles, lectures, retreats, or books. It is important to work with a teacher who has significant meditation experience and a solid understanding of mindfulness practice; who practices what he or she teaches with kindness, compassion, and clear presence; and with whom it is practical to meet on a regular basis.

Join a Community

A more structured way to practice mindfulness is in a group. It can be helpful to join a community as a means to find support, stay connected, and practice together with like-minded people. These communities can be secular or spiritual in nature. You might be able to find a group at your workplace, because many universities and large companies offer wellness programs. These programs invite staff involvement in relaxation or meditation groups or in groups that meet for mindful movement. Many religious traditions also have contemplative practices such as meditation, chant, mantra, and centering prayer as components of their spirituality. Many Hindu, Buddhist, Jewish, Muslim, and Christian communities, for instance, offer groups that meet to practice such contemplative traditions.

Attend Retreats

Taking part in a retreat is one of the most effective ways to deepen one's mindfulness practice. Retreats vary in length, format, and emphasis. Short-term retreats, often held at a university or community space, range from a half day to a weekend in length. Longer retreats, more commonly held in dedicated retreat centers, can be a week or even a month long. Advanced practitioners discuss the benefits of spending months to years in retreat; however, for most practicing clinicians, this amount of time is not an option. Any retreat, no matter the length, provides an opportunity to free oneself from daily obligations, habits, and distractions that may be obstacles to sustained practice. Components of retreats commonly include formal didactic time, discussion time, and time for individual skills-based practice. Just as a music camp enables a person to hone his or her technical skills, a formal meditation retreat serves as an optimal environment for a person to sharpen skills needed for sustained mindfulness practice. A list of retreat centers offering mindfulness-based programs is included in Appendix B at the back of this book.

Informal Practice for the Clinician

In contrast to setting aside time each day as in formal practice, informal practice involves incorporating mindful awareness into activities of daily life and, for the clinician, into clinical work. In essence, a clinician's work and mindfulness practice can, over time, become one and the same. A clinician may use the time spent with and between patients as informal practice. In your work as a clinician, apply intentional moment-to-moment awareness with nonjudgment, openness, and caring. Bring awareness to your patient as well as to your own responses, physical tension, thoughts, and emotions as a means of guiding you in your patient's treatment. Ask the following questions to yourself silently: "Am I in my body? Am I fully present with my patient? Am I in autopilot mode?" Simply asking these questions can bring you back to the present moment.

Practice Grounding (Breathing In and Out) Between Patients (Adapted From Germer et al. 2013, p. 80)

Taking time between appointments can help you to reflect on the patient encounter, clear your mind, and prepare for your next encounter. This reflection can help you be more aware of any residual emotions, content, or countertransference that you carry from session to session. It can also allow you to notice where you hold tension and to release some of this tension through movement or breathing. Taking a mindful moment between patients is a way to enhance your capacity to be fully present with each patient.

- *Instruction*: Schedule 2–3 minutes between patients. Make this a time when you can be alone, without distraction. Consider setting an alarm to avoid worrying about time. Sit in a comfortable chair and close your eyes. Focus attention and awareness on sensations of your body in contact with the chair and your feet on the floor. If you have been sitting for a long period, take this time to practice mindful movement instead. Allow whatever arises in your field of experience to come and go freely. Take note of any sensations in your body, any tension you might be holding. Bring awareness to sensations of the body. Is the quality of the mind clear, cloudy, full of thoughts, or quiet? Notice any residual emotions or thoughts that arise in this moment or thoughts lingering from the previous session. Are there sounds or smells or other sensations that draw your attention? After exploring in silence, bring awareness back to the room. Take a few deep breaths before slowly opening your eyes.

Sit in Silence With Your Patient

Silence can be a compelling means of engaging mindfully with your patient. People often rush to appointments with minds racing or find it difficult to begin talking during the session. Invite your patient to sit in silence with you for

30–60 seconds at the beginning of the session; remind him or her to let go of anything that came before the session or thatis to come. This type of silent awareness of the breath, sensations, emotions, thoughts, and expectations before engaging verbally can help you and your patient meet in a common space.

Communicate Mindfully

Mindful communication means to listen and speak with kindness, compassion, and awareness. In work with patients, clinicians may at times fail to listen with awareness and instead act out of habitual instinct or respond without pausing. Bringing the qualities of openness, nonjudgment, and curiosity to active listening and speaking with patients can be powerful in helping the patient feel heard.

Beckman et al. (2012) assessed the effects that a mindful communication training program had on a group of 70 primary care physicians. A significant percentage of participants "spontaneously reported that learning mindfulness skills improved their capacity to listen more attentively and respond more effectively to others" (p. 816). They attributed the improved communication with patients to the training they received on being in the present moment and listening with curiosity and openness. They also noted that practicing with other physicians helped reduce the feeling of professional isolation.

- *Exercise in mindful listening*: An effective way to practice mindful listening is with a partner. Invite a friend or colleague to join you for this exercise. Designate your partner as person A and yourself as person B. Each person will speak for 2 minutes. To begin, person A tells a story uninterrupted for the full 2 minutes. Person B will listen mindfully to person A without interrupting. Have person B reflect on the following questions while listening and observing how the mind works: "What emotions arise as person A speaks? Do I feel the urge to move or respond in some way while person A speaks? What is the quality of my mind? What thoughts are arising? Do I feel the urge to offer advice or share my own story? Am I making assumptions or judgments while person A speaks?" After person A is finished speaking, take a moment to silently reflect. Both individuals may record thoughts about the interaction and any unspoken observations. Then switch roles so that person B is telling a story for 2 minutes while person A is listening. When person B has completed the story, take a moment to reflect and write down notes. Finally, person A and person B can share their experiences with one another about what it was like to be speaker and listener.

Tips for Practicing Mindful Speaking

- Notice any urges to speak.
- Ask yourself four important questions before speaking: Is it true? Is it kind? Is it helpful? Is it necessary?

- Speak with kind intention, without blaming or condemning.
- Pay attention to nonverbal communication such as tone and body posture.

Tips for Practicing Mindful Listening

- Bring full attention to the person speaking.
- Put away anything that you are working on (e.g., cell phone, pen, paper).
- Remain inquisitive while the other person speaks.
- Maintain attitude of keen interest, openness, and nonjudgment.
- Notice the speaker's response to your full attention.

Practice Single Tasking

Most clinicians value multitasking in an effort to complete work more efficiently. Multitasking implies that a person can simultaneously perform two unconnected tasks. When the tasks are simple, there may be no problem; however, in complex activities, attempts to multitask may result in inadequate performance in one or both tasks (Epstein 2003). There is a growing body of neuroscientific evidence demonstrating that multitasking leads to decreased brain capacity and does not help a person complete tasks more quickly (Ophir et al. 2009). In fact, because multitasking uses additional attentional resources, it can be less efficient overall. Single tasking, in contrast, suggests that a person devotes focused attention to the completion of one activity at a time. It sounds simple, but for most of us who are accustomed to doing several things at once, it can be a challenge. The practice of single tasking is bringing mindfulness to an activity.

Tips for Single Tasking

- Prioritize tasks for the day.
- Focus on one thing at a time until each task is completed.
- Block out specific times during the day to complete patient notes, read e-mail, and make telephone calls.
- Schedule time to eat lunch each day, and during this time, avoid being on the telephone or looking at a screen.
- Notice the urge to multitask throughout the day (e.g., the urge to look at your smartphone while walking).

Challenges and Barriers for Clinician Mindfulness

There are some challenges and barriers in mindfulness practice that are specific to health care clinicians and other universal pitfalls that are experienced to some degree by all practitioners at different points. This section explores these various obstacles as well as their "antidotes." A common theme is that to establish and maintain a consistent practice, we must take a brave and honest look directly at what is getting in the way and allow those obstacles to become our greatest teachers. The way to transcend these obstacles is not by bypassing or going around them but by navigating *through* them via direct engagement with awareness and exploration.

Clinician Barriers

As we clinicians begin to develop a mindfulness practice, we must first face some major paradigm shifts. The first involves a shift from focusing primarily on caring for and attending to others to also include attending to ourselves by focusing inward and caring for ourselves with compassion. The second major shift is from a culture of doing and fixing to that of being and accepting. Furthermore, we must address time constraints and make a strong commitment to practice. We may consider beginning with only 2 minutes a day and allowing that 2 minutes to continue to grow as our practice takes root and blossoms.

Include Your "Self" in Compassion

A commitment to mindfulness is also a commitment to self-care. In our careers as caregivers, we must remember the familiar reminder from the flight attendant: "In the event of an emergency, please put on your own oxygen mask first before assisting others." This guidance to tend to oneself is often forgotten by clinicians, who may consider it antithetical to turn the focus around and begin to practice self-compassion with the same passion given to others. We as clinicians chose the field of caregiving because we felt a calling to help and to heal, and we are rewarded with more praise and recognition the more we give. However, the more passionate we are about giving, the more likely we are to neglect ourselves. Before we know it, we have given our oxygen mask away and are slowly suffocating from burnout, fatigue, and loss of joy and balance, and our relationships begin to suffer. It is at these times that we may be tempted to neglect our mindfulness practice, yet this is precisely the time to fully engage in the practice of radical self-acceptance and self-compassion.

- *Exercise in self-compassion* (adapted from Neff 2012, pp. 79–92): Take a break from your activities. Bring to mind something difficult that recently happened or that may happen soon. First, acknowledge this difficulty by saying something like this to yourself: "This is hard; I'm struggling." Next, remind yourself that this is a universal experience by saying, for example, "Many people are going through tough situations." Finally, bring compassion to your own experience by saying, "May I be kind to myself in this moment." If it feels comfortable, place your hands on your heart. Let feelings of care stream through you. If you find it difficult to let compassion in, imagine telling a friend who is going through a similar situation "I'm here for you" and say this to yourself.

Shift From Doing to Being

Clinician mindfulness practice requires shifting from the biomedical framework of doing to the contemplative framework of being. The "doing mode" seeks to determine what the current state is, what it should be, and what must be done to fix this discrepancy. The "being mode," on the other hand, consists of shifting the frame to simply being present, accepting whatever is occurring in the moment without the need to change it. McCollum and Gehart (2010) point out that both of these modes (doing and being) are necessary for optimal caregiving. They elaborate that mindfulness practice itself can help the clinician to discern when is the right time for doing or being, and how to act on this knowledge. For example, a clinician grounded in mindfulness may choose to sit in silent engagement with a patient who is expressing difficult emotions instead of rushing to act on an impulse to say a comforting statement that may not be as helpful to the patient at the time.

Universal Obstacles: The Five Hindrances and Their Antidotes

Universal obstacles to mindfulness practice include what are termed in Buddhist psychology as *the five hindrances*: restlessness and boredom, sleepiness, doubt, sensory craving, and aversion. The universal antidote is to name the encountered obstacle with loving-kindness, compassion, and the desire to be free of suffering and then gently return back to the practice.

Restlessness and Boredom

The familiar obstacles of restlessness and boredom can pervade one's body and mind. The body may feel jumpy or on edge, with the need to move about or pace. The mind may be planning, making to-do lists, or worrying about patients. A mind in this state cannot be satisfied with things as they are and seeks to escape through distractions such as watching TV. Consider progressive muscle relaxation or using a lying down posture for meditation to calm the body first, and then the mind will follow. If this is still too difficult, consider movement meditation such as walking meditation, Hatha yoga, or tai chi.

Sleepiness

Let's face it: we live in a sleep-deprived society. Many of us notice the minute we slow down long enough to meditate that we become so sleepy that it is difficult to keep our eyes open or our mind focused. Sleepiness can be felt as a heaviness of body and dullness of mind. Discern between true sleep deprivation and resistance to meditation. It is surprising how often our mind tricks us by becoming dull just as we were coming to a breakthrough, experienced as resistance to what is. Ask yourself, "What am I avoiding by falling asleep?" To arouse energy, ensure a steady erect posture, keep eyes (wide) open, splash water on your face, or do a walking or standing meditation.

Doubt

Doubts can arise about many things, such as the mindfulness practice itself, one's life or career, the timing of meditation, or one's body and ability. Doubts may be expressed as worrisome questions: "How do I know what I am doing is right? How do I know if this thing really works and if I am not just wasting my time? What if it takes too long to have any result?" These may be important questions, but they are often asked at the wrong time, such that they interfere with one's practice. It is important to center yourself firmly in the original instructions. After the meditation is over, consider speaking to a trusted wise teacher or seeking relevant readings to enhance faith in the practice.

Sensory Craving

Sensory desire is an attitude of grasping, wanting, pulling, and clinging. When we are stuck in this mindset, we can never be content: "If only I…, then I would be happy, satisfied, enlightened." The here and now is never enough. This attitude stems from a belief that we are not whole, and we seek something from the outside to fill a bottomless pit of desire. This unskillful desire for external stimuli is in contrast to the skillful desire for internal stimuli such as motivation, altruism, and desire for beauty and loving-kindness. When facing sensory craving during meditation, contemplate the impermanence of the desired object or the impermanence of the pleasure derived from it. Reflect on the brevity of life and the fleeting nature of outer satisfaction.

Aversion

Aversion is an attitude of ill will, anger, and irritation toward self, others, or the object of meditation. This attitude closes the heart and condemns. It is the source of tremendous suffering based on dislike of current experience. Negative emotions such as irritation often are not intense but rather insidious and may lead eventually to deep fear or rage. It is crucial to recognize the irritation, allow it to be there, and mindfully choose to either investigate it more deeply or watch as it naturally comes and goes. Long-repressed anger may erupt as rage in meditation and may feel overwhelming and frightening. When ill will toward self or others is noticed, the antidote is to practice loving-kindness, as discussed in the subsection "Universal Antidote: Loving-Kindness," and forgiveness. When fear is noted, this is anticipation of the future. Notice what happens to your beliefs about the world and the future when you are in a state of fear. It is inherent in human nature to want to escape suffering, but trying to get rid of these emotions will not result in less suffering. What we resist tends to persist. Being present with these painful negative emotional states allows us to experience all of life more fully.

Tips for Universal Antidotes to Mindfulness Barriers

- Notice the barrier to mindfulness.
- Name the barrier: "This is boredom." "This is aversion."
- Maintain a beginner's mind. Explore with curiosity and enthusiasm.
- Observe the physical sensations and feel them fully.
- Consider the state of mind: Is it rigid, contracted, flexible, or open?
- Watch these sensations and states arise and allow them to move through you without resisting them or acting on them.
- See what wisdom might be lying beneath the hindrance.
- Contemplate the impermanence of the experience.
- If desired, refocus on your breaths. Count them from 1 to 10.

Universal Antidote: Loving-Kindness

The attitude of loving-kindness, which encompasses feelings of goodwill, kindness, and warmth toward self and others, is a fundamental principle of mindfulness. Practice of loving-kindness is an antidote for many barriers to formal mindfulness, including irritation, anger, and fear, because it opens the heart and allows one's defenses to gently soften.

- *Loving-kindness instruction*: Find a comfortable position. Allow the mind to settle into its natural state by taking some slow deep breaths. Take a moment to acknowledge how things are for you right now, with awareness of your body, your thoughts, your emotions. Bring to mind a dear loved one who easily evokes feelings of warmth and love, possibly a spouse, family member, teacher, or friend. Imagine that the person is present with you. Allow yourself to repeat such phrases as "May you be happy, healthy, joyful, and loved. May you be safe from harm and at peace." You may choose similar phrases that ring true for you. Notice feelings of warmth and love spread through you. When you are ready, shift the focus from your loved one to yourself, repeating these phrases: "May I be happy, healthy, joyful, and loved. May I be safe from harm and at peace." Next, bring to mind a neutral person for whom you do not have strong positive or negative feelings and repeat the original phrases. Then, think of a difficult person with whom you have had some challenges and repeat the phrases. Lastly, repeat these phrases: "May we all be happy, healthy, joyful, and loved. May we all be safe from harm and at peace." Throughout the meditation, notice any resistance and if possible let it go. If the resistance persists, return focus to the loved one and yourself to renew the feeling before returning back to the phrases.

Key Points for Further Study and Reflection

- Developing a mindfulness practice, even if mindfulness is never explicitly taught to patients, is an invaluable tool that will serve to benefit both the clinician (through decreasing factors leading to burnout and stress) and the patient (through enhanced clinician compassion and equanimity and improved patient outcomes).
- Clinicians will benefit from developing formal mindfulness practices, such as sitting or movement-based meditation, as well as informal practices such as using mindfulness during daily activities, including during and between patient sessions.
- There are several universal obstacles and barriers to practicing mindfulness, as well as some barriers that apply specifically to clinicians. These can be addressed in various ways, but the practice of loving-kindness can serve as a universal antidote.

References

Beckman HB, Wendland M, Mooney C, et al: The impact of a program in mindful communication on primary care physicians. Acad Med 87(6):815–819, 2012 22534599

Davis DM, Hayes JA: What are the benefits of mindfulness? A practice review of psychotherapy-related research. Psychotherapy (Chic) 48(2):198–208, 2011 21639664

Epstein RM: Mindful practice in action, I: technical competence, evidence-based medicine, and relationship-centered care. Fam Syst Health 21(1):1–9, 2003

Germer CK, Siegel RD, Fulton PR (eds): Mindfulness and Psychotherapy, 2nd Edition. New York, Guilford, 2013

Irving JA, Dobkin PL, Park J: Cultivating mindfulness in health care professionals: a review of empirical studies of mindfulness-based stress reduction (MBSR). Complement Ther Clin Pract 15(2):61–66, 2009 19341981

Kornfield J: A Path With Heart: A Guide Through the Perils and Promises of Spiritual Life. New York, Bantam, 1993

Krasner MS, Epstein RM, Beckman H, et al: Association of an educational program in mindful communication with burnout, empathy, and attitudes among primary care physicians. JAMA 302(12):1284–1293, 2009 19773563

McCollum EE, Gehart DR: Using mindfulness meditation to teach beginning therapists therapeutic presence: a qualitative study. J Marital Fam Ther 36(3):347–360, 2010 20618581

Neff KD: The science of self-compassion, in Compassion and Wisdom in Psychotherapy. Edited by Germer CK, Siegel RD. New York, Guilford, 2012, pp 79–92

Ophir E, Nass C, Wagner AD: Cognitive control in media multitaskers. Proc Natl Acad Sci USA 106(37):15,583–15,587, 2009 19706386

Shapiro SL, Carlson LE: The Art and Science of Mindfulness: Integrating Mindfulness Into Psychology and the Helping Professions. Washington, DC, American Psychological Association, 2009

5

Mindfulness in Practice

Incorporating Mindfulness Inside and Outside of Sessions

Jonathan Kaplan, Ph.D.
Doris F. Chang, Ph.D.

We should be blessed if we lived in the present always, and took advantage of every accident that befell us, like the grass which confesses the influence of the slightest dew that falls on it; and did not spend our time in atoning for the neglect of past opportunities, which we call doing our duty. We loiter in winter while it is already spring.

Henry David Thoreau, *Walden*

IN THIS CHAPTER we provide practical guidelines for how to create and customize mindfulness practices for your patients. We present a conceptual model to guide your integration of mindfulness, which can be used within a variety of theoretical frameworks, including psychodynamic, cognitive-behavioral, and integrative approaches. Using this model, we provide specific practices that can be implemented both inside and outside of sessions. In addition, we discuss the various challenges that may arise when establishing a mindfulness practice and provide ways to overcome them. Finally, to make the model and practices more understandable, we provide a case example describing how they were used with a particular patient.

Mindfulness has become increasingly popular over the past few decades. During the year 1981, no research studies were published with "mindfulness" in the title. Eight studies were published in 1990, only 22 were released in 2000, and 674 were published in 2015 (Black 2016). The growth of scientific interest in mindfulness has been mirrored by its increased visibility in the popular media. In 2015, *Time* magazine heralded the "mindfulness revolution." Celebrities such as Oprah Winfrey, Arianna Huffington, Deepak Chopra, Kobe Bryant, and Anderson Cooper have all touted its benefits. Although the preponderance of clinical research findings and anecdotal reports provide strong evidence that mindfulness can be helpful in enhancing wellness and life satisfaction, many other activities, including exercise, also have benefits. Thus, when considering the introduction of mindfulness into psychotherapy with a particular patient, the first question to consider is "Why?"

The "Fit" of Mindfulness

To assess the appropriateness of mindfulness as a therapeutic approach for a patient, it is important to consider three factors: purpose, practice, and person (Kaplan 2014). By keeping these factors in mind, you can tailor your approach to your particular patient and evaluate its effectiveness over time.

Purpose

Studies investigating a variety of mindfulness practices have documented their health-promoting benefits, including reduced anxiety, improved attention and concentration, reduced stress, improved physical functioning, and faster recovery from illness. Practitioners of mindfulness have also observed that it allows them to be more present, live in the moment, be less distracted, and act with greater awareness and intention. In our own work as therapists, we have noticed that mindfulness can be clinically useful for patients in five key ways:

- By increasing awareness of some pattern, experience, or issue
- By promoting relaxation
- By cultivating acceptance of some mental or emotional experience
- By developing insight into an unconscious process
- By facilitating the capacity to choose a more effective response

It is helpful to consider these potential benefits when exploring the suitability of mindfulness practice for a particular patient. As part of this consideration, it is important to contemplate, "What particular outcome do I hope my patient will achieve or develop?"

Practice

Mindfulness constitutes paying attention kindly to whatever arises moment to moment in immediate experience. As such, there are many ways to cultivate this awareness and a plethora of things to notice. You are limited only by your creativity in determining what might be the best initial practice for your patient. To help you sort through these options, we include seven considerations suggested by Pollack et al. (2014):

1. **Emphasis on concentration, open awareness, or acceptance-based techniques:** Would it be better for your patient to practice focusing repeatedly on one specific object; closely follow his or her wandering mind; or cultivate compassion, loving-kindness, or another contemplative state of mind?
2. **Informal, formal, or retreat practice:** Is it helpful for your patient to practice "on the go" in daily life, to practice through formal meditation, or to attend a meditation retreat?
3. **Coarse or subtle objects of attention:** Is the object of attention easy for the patient to notice, such as sound or an obvious physical sensation (e.g., feet touching the ground), or harder to discern (e.g., the passage of air across the area between the nostrils and upper lip)?
4. **Religious or secular approach:** If your patient is religious, then he or she might like to explore mindfulness from the perspective of his or her tradition. Although typically associated with Buddhism, mindfulness has parallels in all religions. Alternatively, you can maintain a secular focus in practice.
5. **Attention to nonprovocative objects or problematic areas:** Would it be preferable for your patient to note "safe" areas of experience or to attend to ones that are more challenging, such as difficult emotions or schemas?

6. **Narrative or experiential focus:** Do you encourage your patient to talk about his or her story or to rest in moment-to-moment experience?
7. **Focus on relative or absolute truth:** Mindfulness can facilitate profound spiritual awakening. Do you encourage your patient to pursue mindfulness deeply in this way or, more commonly, to seek more conventional insight?

We add the following three additional issues to contemplate in considering which mindfulness approaches are most suitable for your patient:

1. **Physically active or sedate:** Would it be more helpful for your patient to practice mindfulness while sitting, standing, lying down, or moving?
2. **Internal or external focus:** Although all experiences ultimately are processed internally, the object of focus might be an internal experience (e.g., a physical sensation or thought) or might reside outside of the body (e.g., a sound or a picture).
3. **Physical, mental, or emotional awareness:** If your patient focuses attention on internal experiences, is it preferable to note physical sensations, thoughts, or feelings?

No one particular practice is the best starting point for introducing mindfulness to your patients. If you are unsure of where to begin, we have found it helpful to start with a seated, secular, concentration-based practice focused on a coarse, nonprovocative, internal, physical experience—in other words, mindfulness of breathing.

Person

Many people assume that mindfulness can be beneficial for everyone, yet it is important to recognize that mindfulness might not be the best fit for a specific patient. Depending on the patient's goal, another practice might be more effective. For example, if your patient wants to relax, then physical exercise, massage, or biofeedback might be more effective. Taken further, it is also possible that mindfulness may be counterproductive given the patient's current struggles or problems.

In our experience, there are three problem areas—trauma, psychosis, and severe depression— that deserve careful consideration. Because mindfulness practice has an emphasis on the body, this practice can be particularly difficult or provocative for people who have a trauma history. For patients experiencing hallucinations, the silence characteristic of mindfulness exercises can increase susceptibility to attend to the hallucinations. When people are actively experiencing delusions or deeply held depressive thoughts, mindfulness exercises (especially meditation) can increase paranoia or intensify the depression. In such circumstances, it is difficult for those individuals to simply note "thoughts as thoughts." Instead, they are prone to get caught up in thinking about their worries and fears and to relate to their thoughts as real and personal, which can heighten distress. The ability to focus and maintain attention on a neutral object cannot compete with these more provocative prompts.

Accordingly, it is important to exercise caution when introducing mindfulness to patients who suffer from these conditions, particularly when you are relatively new to mindfulness practice yourself. If you do decide to introduce it, then we recommend that you teach a grounding technique beforehand, such as a mantra-based meditation or body awareness focused on simple movement (e.g., pushing feet into the ground). This will help "build the attention muscle" and provide a neutral stimulus if the experience becomes too overwhelming for the patient.

Once you determine the reason(s) for introducing mindfulness, you might consider implementing a system to track its effectiveness. Mindfulness measures, such as the Mindfulness Attention Awareness Scale (Brown and Ryan 2003) and the Five Facet Mindfulness Questionnaire (Baer et al. 2006), can provide an overall indication of a patient's level of awareness in different situations, whereas other measures might be more focused on the specific treatment goal(s).

Case Example

Judy, a 30-year-old single woman, was interested in practicing mindfulness to "feel better" and get some relief from her feelings of anxiety and low self-esteem. Instead of "quick-fix" strategies, she wanted something that could bring about profound personal change. She was willing to practice mindfulness meditation but had difficulty focusing on her breath. She would become tense and frequently wondered whether she was "doing it right." Although she could have simply observed these reactions, she was becoming increasingly frustrated and was poised to "give up" on the practice. In response, the clinician invited her to switch her mindfulness practice to sound, which she found to be easier and more relaxing. Judy spent 10 minutes each day simply listening and noticing what she could hear. She would acknowledge the sound and its apparent location, as well as her mind's tendency to ascribe it as coming from a particular source (e.g., an ambulance). She was unwilling to fill out detailed surveys that assessed her anxiety, stress, or level of mindfulness; however, she was willing to maintain a basic log of her practices. She noted the specific practice, the duration, and a simplified assessment of her overall mood for the day as indicated by a ☺, ☹, or ☺.

Conceptual Overview of Practice: SPARK Model

There are many ways to practice mindfulness. One can breathe mindfully, eat mindfully, commute mindfully, bathe mindfully, listen mindfully, meditate mindfully, and so on. To elucidate the processes involved in cultivating mindfulness, we have developed a transtheoretical approach, the SPARK model, which identifies five distinct stages of mindfulness: Stopping (or Slowing Down), Perceiving, Allowing, Reflecting, and Knowing.[1] This model provides a teaching framework for developing practices that are tailored to the needs and capabilities of a particular patient. You can also share the model with patients once they develop the appropriate insight to craft their own practices.

Stopping (or Slowing Down)

Mindfulness can develop only when we *stop* (or *slow down*) our usual way of operating in the world. Typically, we are lost in thought, too immersed in an activity (e.g., watching TV), or dividing our attention among multiple tasks, and we do not notice much else. Mindfulness, then, invites us to relate to our experiences in ways that are attentive, curious, and kind. To do so, we need to make a conscious effort to stop or slow what we are doing. Once we have done so, we are in a position to bring sustained awareness to some aspect of experience. In your therapy with patients, you can make a deliberate shift to conducting a mindfulness exercise together (e.g., leading a meditation) or periodically inviting your patient to check in with his or her sensory experiences (e.g., noting physical sensations in the body), reflecting on what he or she observes, and then continue your discussion.

Perceiving

The initial application of mindfulness involves the act of perceiving. We tune into some aspect of our immediate experience and make an effort to maintain that awareness over time. At this stage, we can pay attention to many different aspects of experience, such as noticing what we see, feel, hear, taste, and smell.

---

[1] Readers might be familiar with RAIN as an acronym for **R**ecognize, **A**ccept, **I**nvestigate, and **N**onidentify, often used to address difficult emotions. Although RAIN is useful, we prefer the SPARK model for several reasons: 1) it avoids the connotation of passivity associated with the word *acceptance*, 2) it encourages inquiry without any predetermined conclusions, and 3) it recognizes that nonidentification is just one possible effect of mindfulness practice and reflection.

Additionally, we are able to observe our thoughts, emotions, behaviors, and intention. The specific object of attention will vary, depending on what you think will be most beneficial for your patient.

The predominant attitude is one of curiosity. Patients are encouraged to be engaged and interested in whatever arises in each moment. For example, if a patient is paying attention to breathing, then he or she might notice that a particular breath is short and shallow. What about the next one? What will it be like? The patient is encouraged to discover inquisitively what is unfolding in real time.

Allowing

The *allowing* stage of mindfulness practice is critical. Indeed, we consider it to be the most helpful aspect of initial practice. Patients are encouraged to adopt a kind, accepting attitude toward whatever they observe. Allowing whatever they are experiencing to be present can be difficult, especially in the case of painful sensations, unwanted thoughts, traumatic memories, or hurtful emotions. At such times, we encourage patients to make room for these unpleasant experiences, as well as their aversive reactions. If it is helpful, they can greet their observations openly by repeating phrases such as "yes," "hello," "welcome," or "it's OK that...." In this way, they can cultivate an attitude to accept the negative experience and their rejection to its presence.

Reflecting

If your patient is interested in mindfulness as a means of developing insight into his or her mind, personality, relationships, or the world, then it is necessary to invite purposeful reflection on the patient's experience. *Reflecting* is the process of asking questions about what is being observed and experienced. At this stage, you are welcome to introduce forms of questioning that are specific to your theoretical orientation or centered on the phenomenological experience itself. For example, if a patient describes perceiving a strong sensation in his or her body, you can invite the patient to consider questions such as, "What is this?" "What does this feeling want me to know?" "Is this me?" or "How do I understand this?" If your patient notes a persistent thought or belief, you can help the patient reflect on questions such as, "How old is this thought?" "Who does this thought remind me of?" or "Is this who I am?"

Again, it is important to be sensitive to each patient's skill level and stability of attention. In the initial stages of mindfulness practice, inquiry regarding one's perceptions is discouraged because it can produce ruminative or overly intellectualized responses. However, once a degree of quietude is achieved through the initial practice, guiding the patient to reflect on what he or she observes can have profound effects on how the patient brings the practice forward in other aspects of his or her life. Mindfulness can open the door to a greater understanding of oneself or even profound religious or spiritual insights.

Knowing

Knowing represents the outcome of the reflecting process. On the basis of your patient's inquiry into his or her internal experiences, various "truths" emerge that reflect levels of profundity and emotional resonance that are often not achieved through normal conversation or intellectual consideration. What emerges is an *embodied knowing* of some profound truth that allows your patient greater agency and freedom. It is similar to how we, as adults, know that we will get burned if we touch a hot stove. We no longer need to consciously remind ourselves not to touch the stove—we experience this knowledge as truth and live accordingly. Practicing mindfulness in this way can be profoundly life changing.

Case Example *(continued)*

Recently, after a mindfulness meditation, Judy noted that she had considerable trouble concentrating on sound and that she was lost in thoughts about her job, partner, dinner, and exercise regimen. Invited to make sense of that experience, she noted insightfully, "My mind is always on!" With that observation, she realized that she did not need to take her thoughts so seriously. Just like having the TV on all day, she didn't always need to pay attention to what is on. Sometimes, the programming isn't particularly interesting or meaningful.

Practice Inside of Sessions

In your sessions, we advise you to incorporate mindfulness practice both formally—through guided meditations—and informally—through periodic check-ins of your patient's sensory experience. In a session, you have a precious opportunity to guide your patient in specific exercises grounded in your expert assessment of his or her history, needs, resources, and capabilities. You can then debrief the experience to promote the patient's insight, answer questions, and address particular obstacles. Recording your in-session guided meditations and making them available to your patient offers much more personalization and may promote greater transferability to the home environment than prerecorded meditations may offer.

Formal Exercises

Using the SPARK model and your initial consideration of what kinds of practices will be most helpful, you can guide your patients through mindfulness meditations. Your ability to lead your patients in mindfulness activities will be significantly influenced by your personal experience of the practice. As a result, we strongly recommend that you cultivate your own mindfulness practice through meditation, certification courses, and retreat experiences.

For beginners to mindfulness, we typically suggest starting with hearing sound or feeling physical sensations (e.g., breathing) in the body. Generally speaking, these perceptions are easier to notice and less likely than other perceptions to promote rumination. For many patients, mindfulness of difficult emotions is an especially fruitful practice (see sample script below). However, it requires that your patient be able to concentrate for discrete periods of time and purposefully shift awareness to different objects. Cultivation of these abilities comes with practice. As you and your patient work toward expanding the object of his or her attention, it is important to be aware of any desired goals and accept whatever arises in experience. In fact, there is an inherent contradiction here: whereas your patient practices mindfulness to achieve some end result, mindfulness encourages him or her to accept reality and experience as it is, without any expectation that it should be otherwise. In this way, having an implicit agenda for change runs counter to the attitudinal foundation of the practice. This contradiction is inevitable, especially in the beginning. Without any motivation for change, there will be no investment in actual practice. It is important to hold this intention lightly, however, and recognize if and when it becomes more problematic as your patient's practice matures.

Sample script for mindfulness of difficult emotions

Please find a comfortable position that prompts you to feel both relaxed and alert. Take a few deep breaths, feeling your stomach and chest rise as you breathe in and fall as you breathe out. If you feel safe, I'd ask that you close your eyes because it will make it easier to focus on your feelings. Alternatively, you can keep your eyes open, while gazing down toward the floor.

[Pause]

In this exercise, I'll invite you to focus on your emotions. To begin, I'd like for you to recall a specific incident that caused strong emotional reactions in as much detail as you can. When exactly did this happen? Where were you? Were you alone or with other people? What actually occurred? What did you do or say? What were you feeling?

Sample script for mindfulness of difficult emotions *(continued)*

[You might ask the person to actually speak the answers to these questions aloud. The purpose in starting with this contemplation is to prompt your patient to experience a difficult emotion. If the patient already has a strong, uncomfortable feeling when you begin the exercise, you can skip the recollection of the event and proceed to the exploration of the embodied emotion.]

Now, I'd like for you to move your attention away from remembering the event to how you're feeling right now…in this moment. What are you feeling now?

[Check in with your patient to ensure that he or she is feeling a reasonably strong, difficult emotion reminiscent of his or her triggering event. If not, you can continue guiding a recollection of the event to prompt a reaction or switch to a general body scan.]

So, right now, as you sit here in this space, you're feeling [emotion]. Where do you feel that emotion most prominently in your body?

[Once your patient has identified a strong physical sensation associated with that emotion, then you can proceed to ask the following questions, pausing after each one. As you hear your patient's answers, see if you can imagine feeling it yourself.]

What does it feel like? Where specifically can you feel it? Can you show me the edges of it with your finger? Does it feel hot or cold? Does it feel deep in your body or more toward the surface of your skin? Does it have a dynamic quality—is it moving in some way—or does it feel static?

[Prompted by these questions, your patient will focus his or her attention more closely on the physical feeling arising with that emotion. Often, the simple act of resting awareness on the sensation will cause it to subside. If, however, the sensation persists, you can ask your patient to bring explicit acceptance to the process of noticing.]

Now, I'd like for you to introduce a kind, welcoming attitude toward what you're experiencing right now. In your mind, I'd like for you to say, "Yes" or "It's OK that…" relative to whatever you notice. For example, you might think to yourself, "Yes, I feel tension in my chest" or "Yes, it feels hot." Please continue to provide this explicit permission for your observations, including your own reactions and judgments. For example, you might think, "Yes, I don't like this," or "Yes, this is painful," or "Yes, I was thinking of something else."

[Allow your patient to continue in this way for another 5 minutes.]

Now, I'd like for you to release this focus on the feeling and start bringing your attention back to the room. Initially, you can take note of the sounds in the room. Then, notice the temperature of the air on your skin. And, whenever you're ready, you can open your eyes and return with your full presence and awareness.

Most people expect that they will be able to pay attention dutifully during a mindfulness activity. However, as we know, attention waxes and wanes. Although unwavering attention might be their intention, it is more important for your patients to examine how they speak to themselves when they notice that their awareness has shifted. It is crucial to extend that attitude of kindness and acceptance to the inevitable wandering of attention, too.

Informal Exercises

In addition to using formal guided experiences, you can facilitate the development of mindfulness via more informal practices, such as inviting your patient to check in periodically with his or her sensory experience. Often, therapy can be quite cerebral and emotional, and we find it beneficial to cultivate a patient's ability to shift attention and consider other sources of sensory information as equally valid. For example, when introducing patients to mindfulness, we often invite them to close their eyes and describe the room—the objects, colors, placement, and so on. This can often be quite humbling for patients, especially when they have been having sessions in the same room for a while. They commonly do not even know the color of the sofa they have been sitting on for weeks. Similarly, at any point, you can invite your patients to describe what they hear—making a distinction between the sound itself and the mind's tendency to ascribe it to a particular source (e.g., *rrrr* vs. a truck idling) or imbue it with particular meaning (e.g., "that is an annoying sound"). We often ask patients to check in with physical feelings in the body, especially when they are experiencing an intense emotion. If your patients are eating or drinking in session, you can playfully ask them to describe what they taste. All of these prompts are inviting your patients to become more observant about their sensory perceptions of their internal and external world.

At the risk of confusing you with another acronym, we introduce a way of conducting a mindful "check-in." In any moment, you can direct your patient to attend to any of the following GATES of experience:

- **Goals:** What is important or necessary that I do right now? What do I need? What do I want? In this moment, what is my goal or intention?
- **Actions:** What am I actually doing right now? Specifically, am I walking? Sitting? Standing? Reading? Watching TV? Texting? Waiting? Perhaps I am doing a few things simultaneously? It is easy for judgment to intrude here (e.g., "I am wasting time"), so be as objective as possible about identifying the behavior in which you are engaged.
- **Thoughts:** What is going through my mind? What was I just thinking about? Resist the urge to simply label it as "nothing." When we are con-

scious, we are always thinking about something. Our minds are never blank. We might consider what is coming to mind as not particularly important or insightful, yet we are still thinking about something.

- **Emotions:** What am I feeling emotionally? Happy? Sad? Angry? Bored? Sometimes, people have a difficult time identifying how they feel. Accordingly, you might use a list of emotions to help patients distinguish them. If you don't want to (or can't) be so specific about your emotional experience, an alternative is to indicate the valence of what you are feeling. Right now, are you having a pleasant, unpleasant, or neutral feeling? Emotionally, would you rate your current state using "thumbs up," "thumbs down," or "thumbs sideways?"
- **Senses:** What information am I perceiving through my five senses? In this particular moment, what do I see? Hear? Taste? Smell? Touch? You might deepen this awareness by breaking down particular observations into more discrete perceptions. With sight, for example, you can attend to color, form, reflection, shading, and other visual cues. With taste, you can access the texture of food or drink, as well as the flavors of bitter, sour, salty, sweet, and umami.

These prompts to be mindful of different dimensions of experience share some commonalities with the monitoring activities commonly used in cognitive-behavioral therapy. Thought records, used to help patients identify their cognitive, affective, and physiological responses to triggering events, also can be used to support patients' development of mindfulness. Tracking their mood throughout the day can also help patients to notice how mood fluctuates naturally. However, a mindfulness approach goes beyond these traditional monitoring activities to widen the focus to include more neutral as well as positive experiences, with the goal of helping patients become more attuned to the dynamic nature of their minds and bodies. In addition to tracking mood, mindfulness also provides a framework for patients to practice observing their experiences and interpretations from a distance, by actively encouraging a kind, nonjudgmental stance.

More relationally oriented psychodynamic therapists may also find some similarities between the GATES model and relational interventions used to explore transference and countertransference reactions in session. Cultivating patients' mindful awareness can help support this relational work while calling attention to the patients' perceptions of self and other as perceptions and not the thing itself.

Improving Your Ability to Lead Mindfulness Practices

As discussed in Chapter 4, "Practice What You Preach," the best ways to improve as a mindfulness teacher are through dedicated personal practice combined with expert supervision. We encourage you to try many different mindfulness exercises and meditations, led by different teachers. In this way, you will come to realize the diversity of voices in the mindfulness world while exploring what fits best with your own teaching style and preferences. Further, we recommend that you find ways to receive constructive feedback on how you lead mindfulness exercises. For example, you can enroll in a program for meditation teacher training, pursue certification in Mindfulness-Based Stress Reduction, hire a local meditation expert to provide supervision, or even create a group of like-minded peers and practice with each other. As you try out different approaches and find your voice as a teacher, you may find your practice preferences and training needs changing over time. This is perfectly fine. In fact, your practice is likely to inform what and how you teach. Trust in the process.

Practice Outside of Sessions

Once you have introduced your patient to mindfulness through in-session instruction and practice, collaborate with him or her to develop a plan for practice outside of the session. Practice can be formal or informal, depending on your patient's level of commitment and available resources. As with any type of therapeutic goal setting, exploring your patient's priorities, needs, and concerns will help the two of you develop a tailored and feasible plan for practice. Ongoing monitoring of the patient's extratherapy practice and its effects is recommended so that you can update or revise the plan as the patient's needs change.

Formal Practice

In structuring a formal mindfulness practice with a patient, we typically explore the following guidelines as a starting point for discussion:

1. **Practice at a regular time every day.** This can be based on clock time (e.g., 8:00 A.M.) or a daily event (e.g., in the morning after walking the dog). Deciding ahead of time *when* the patient will practice mindfulness and inserting the practice into his or her daily schedule is a crucial part of developing the habit. Explore with your patient the optimal time for his or her daily practice.
2. **Specify a concrete goal for the type and duration of daily mindfulness practice.** Would your patient benefit initially from more body-based practices such as mindfulness of breath or a body scan? Should the patient practice for 5, 10, 15, or 30 minutes a day?
3. **Obtain appropriate written scripts or recordings of guided meditations.** Provide your patient with written copies of helpful scripts (for self-guided meditations), copies of your own in-session recordings, or links to freely

available digital downloads. Our Web site, www.sohocbt.com, includes recordings that patients can download for their use. We also recommend the recordings posted on the Web sites of key meditation research centers (e.g., the UCLA Mindful Awareness Research Center) and of popular teachers and authors (e.g., Sharon Salzberg, Jack Kornfield, and Tara Brach). Some useful resources are listed in Appendix B at the back of this book.

4. **Obtain any additional material supports that are needed.** Explore what additional material resources are needed to support your patient's out-of-session practice goals. Does the patient have a quiet place to practice where he or she will not be disturbed? Does the patient prefer a seated meditation but not have an appropriate cushion? Does the patient enjoy guided meditations but need to fix his or her CD player or figure out how to download the MP3s to a device? Does the patient need to get a pair of headphones so as not to disturb others? Discuss strategies for addressing each of the material needs identified by your patient.

5. **Obtain any interpersonal supports that are needed.** In our experience, it can be extremely helpful for beginning meditators to participate in a regular meditation group. A patient might choose a group organized by a local meditation center, organize a group (e.g., a lunchtime meditation group at work), or join a virtual group that exists online. Even texting brief notes about daily practice to a mindfulness buddy (e.g., "July 1, 15 min., mindfulness of breath) can provide encouragement and promote accountability.

6. **Consider using technology to help.** Besides the vast library of resources on mindfulness available online, many patients enjoy using meditation apps created for smartphones and other devices (see Appendix B at the back of this book). Many apps provide useful content, such as guided meditations; track frequency and duration of each meditation session; and connect the user to an online community of meditators. Some of these apps are free, whereas others require a monthly subscription.

7. **Consider attending a meditation retreat.** As mindfulness becomes increasingly popular and is packaged alongside other wellness activities, such as yoga, many patients may express interest in attending a meditation retreat. It is difficult to prepare your patient for the retreat experience if you have not personally attended a retreat yourself. Some retreat centers are explicitly connected to a specific religious tradition; others are more secular in their approach. Some require a signed release for individuals who have a history of mental illness, confirming that they are under the care of a mental health provider who may be contacted if the individuals become symptomatic while on retreat. Research the different options in your local area so that you can properly advise your patient if he or she is interested in going on a retreat. (Some retreat centers are listed in Appendix B at the back of this book.)

Informal Practice

In addition to, or instead of, engaging in a formal mindfulness practice outside of the session, patients also benefit from cultivating mindfulness through more informal activities. For example, patients who find it comforting to be with their pets may set an intention to spend 10 minutes each evening mindfully petting their cat or dog, focusing on the sensory experiences (touch, sight, scent, and hearing) and their responses. As noted earlier, informal practices can extend to mindful eating, commuting, and even e-mailing. Collaborate with each patient to identify an informal mindfulness activity or range of activities to do out of session that allow for regular, daily practice. We also recommend exploring the issues raised in the previous subsection on formal practice regarding an appropriate time, setting, activity type, and duration of practice, as well as the resources and supports needed.

Obstacles

It is not uncommon for patients to describe difficulties initiating and maintaining a mindfulness practice program outside of sessions. Obstacles to mindfulness practice are likely to fall into three categories: mental, circumstantial, and lifestyle issues. In our experience, most difficulties that arise in practicing mindfulness are produced by the mind—for example, generating difficult mental conditions for practice (e.g., restlessness or sleepiness), forgetting to practice, or procrastinating. Although there are several classical Buddhist "antidotes" to difficulties that arise in the mind, our best advice is to help your patient adopt a gentle curiosity about the obstacle itself. For example, if your patient becomes sleepy or restless when practicing mindfulness, the patient can investigate where that feeling resides in the body or reflect on the conditions that give rise to that quality of mind.

Sometimes, there are objectively difficult circumstances that interfere with practice. For example, it might be hard to meditate at work if a person does not have a private, quiet place. In such circumstances, your patient can either decide to practice elsewhere (or at a different time) or flexibly adapt the practice to the circumstances. It will be necessary to remind your patient to hold expectations for practice lightly: meditating on the subway is going to be very different from meditating at home, for example. And, regardless of the experience itself, following through on the intention to practice will help cultivate crucial attitudinal components of mindfulness, including acceptance, kindness, openness, and curiosity.

Finally, your patient's lifestyle choices might make it difficult to maintain a regular practice. Within Buddhism, there is considerable emphasis on ethical behavior that does not harm oneself or others. The advice includes abstaining from drugs and alcohol, communicating truthfully and kindly, and avoiding certain occupations. The reason for these prescriptions is not that drugs and alcohol, lying, criticizing, and working in certain professions are inherently wrong, bad, or evil. Instead, the Buddhist texts describe these factors as readily interfering with one's ability to cultivate a wholesome state of mind. Lying, for example, can create anxiety and rumination about being discovered. Similarly, an evening of drinking alcohol or using drugs often leads to a less focused and clear mind the next day. In such circumstances, you can wonder aloud about possible connections between these behaviors and difficulties in practice that your patient is experiencing. Then, you can invite the patient to notice if there is any connection between his or her actions and subsequent mindfulness practice. Again, the purpose is not to place a value judgment on the behavior as good or bad but rather to notice its relationship to cultivating mindfulness and adjust future actions and expectations accordingly.

Case Example *(continued)*

Judy had been meditating regularly and experiencing lighter moods relative to her practice. However, during a busy time at work, she stopped practicing and found it difficult to restart. Her mind regularly told her that she did not have time, and she thought that it would "not count" if she could meditate for only a few minutes. Once she recognized the ways in which her mind was tricking her (and noted the improved mood reflected in her daily logs), she resumed meditating for a few minutes a day and soon reestablished her practice.

Revisiting the Effectiveness of Mindfulness

Once your patient has been practicing mindfulness regularly and using a variety of methods, it becomes appropriate to ask this question: Which practices have helped this particular person achieve his or her stated purpose?

Ultimately, the evidence in favor of incorporating mindfulness—or not—will emerge from your patient's experience of it. The proof is in the "patient pudding," so to speak. From your observations and analysis, you will help your patient realize the benefits of practice. From here, you can provide periodic reminders and encouragement to maintain the patient's practice or revisit it whenever necessary.

Key Points for Further Study and Reflection

- To assess the appropriateness of integrating mindfulness into psychotherapy, it is important to consider the fit between the purpose underlying the decision; the specific practice(s) that you will employ; and the personal characteristics of your patient.
- Providing conceptual guidance for your mindfulness practice, the SPARK model incorporates five processes: **S**topping (or slowing down), **P**erceiving, **A**llowing, **R**eflecting, and **K**nowing.
- Mindfulness practice can occur both inside and outside of sessions and can be formal (e.g., meditation) or informal (e.g., mindful eating).
- Obstacles will naturally arise in mindfulness practice. Be patient and explore various ways to overcome them.

References

Baer RA, Smith GT, Hopkins J, et al: Using self-report assessment methods to explore facets of mindfulness. Assessment 13(1):27–45, 2006 16443717

Black D: Mindfulness journal publications by year: 1980–2015. Pasadena, CA, American Mindfulness Research Association, 2016. Available at: https://goamra.org/wp-content/uploads/2014/05/trends_AMRA_2016.png. Accessed July 13, 2016.

Brown KW, Ryan RM: The benefits of being present: mindfulness and its role in psychological well-being. J Pers Soc Psychol 84(4):822–848, 2003 12703651

Kaplan J: When mindfulness training doesn't work. Advances in Cognitive Therapy Newsletter 15(1):4, 2014

Pollack SM, Pedulla T, Siegel RD: Sitting Together: Essential Skills for Mindfulness-Based Psychotherapy. New York, Guilford, 2014

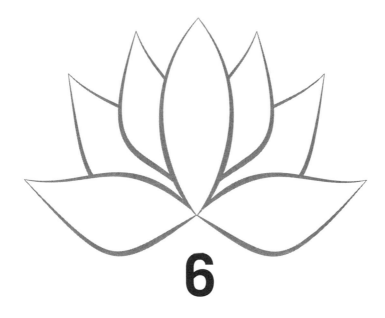

6

Mindfulness as an Intervention in the Treatment of Psychopathology

Sarah Zoogman, Ph.D.
Elizabeth Foskolos, M.A.
Eleni Vousoura, Ph.D.

[S]ymptoms of illness or distress, plus your feelings about them, can be viewed as messengers coming to give you important and useful information about your body or about your mind.... Our real challenge when we have symptoms is to see if we can listen to their messages and really hear them and take them to heart, that is, make the connection fully.

Jon Kabat-Zinn, *Full Catastrophe Living*

MINDFULNESS PRACTICE has long been regarded as a valuable tool promoting wellness among generally healthy individuals. In more recent years, mindfulness has further emerged as a clinical intervention for helping people who suffer from mental illness. The clinical application of mindfulness is most commonly described as *mindfulness-based intervention* (MBI), an umbrella term to denote treatments that are guided by mindfulness principles underlying Buddhism and other religious and spiritual practices and that focus on the self-regulation of attention in the moment and in a nonjudgmental and accepting way. Despite originating from spiritual practices, MBIs are secular, clinically based methods that are embedded in manual-based psychotherapeutic protocols. MBIs are rapidly growing in popularity, and over the past decade, there is an ever-increasing implementation of mindfulness training programs targeting a range of clinical disorders across diverse patient populations.

Accumulating evidence demonstrates the efficacy of MBIs in targeting a variety of common mental disorders, including depression, anxiety, and pain-related disorders, and mounting evidence shows their promise in targeting trauma-related disorders, attention-deficit/hyperactivity disorder (ADHD), severe mental illness, disordered eating, and addictive behaviors. Much less is known, however, about the specific ways in which mindfulness brings about change. A solid understanding of these *mechanisms of therapeutic change* is crucial for practitioners to tailor their interventions to individual clients, increase the ecological validity of these interventions, and optimize their therapeutic impact.

The primary goal of this chapter is to bring together, in an operative and understanding way, the theoretical and empirical knowledge on the clinical application of mindfulness in the treatment of psychopathology. More specifically, this chapter aims to inform the reader about the core principles and strategies of MBIs in the treatment of specific mental disorders; to review available empirical evidence on the effectiveness of these interventions across different mental disorders; and to advocate for the need to hone our understanding of how mindfulness works in order to deliver more personalized care to our patients, tailored to their unique problems and treatment needs.

Mindfulness-Based Interventions for Specific Disorders

The past few decades have witnessed a proliferation of MBIs targeting a wide range of mental disorders in a variety of populations. Before embarking on a thorough review of the implementation of mindfulness in mental health, we need to distinguish between psychosocial interventions that integrate mindfulness into their core structure, such as Mindfulness-Based Stress Reduction (MBSR) and Mindfulness-Based Cognitive Therapy (MBCT), and interventions that use mindfulness among other therapeutic strategies, such as dialectical behavior therapy (DBT) and acceptance and commitment therapy (ACT). This chapter focuses solely on mindfulness-based treatments because blended interventions such as DBT and ACT differ significantly from pure MBIs with regard to their definition of mindfulness techniques, as well as the format and structure of their mindfulness module. Each mindfulness intervention covered in this chapter is described in Table 6–1. In the following subsections, we discuss the use of mindfulness-based treatments for various mental disorders.

Depression and Suicidality

Depression is a highly prevalent and debilitating condition characterized by sadness, loss of interest, low self-esteem or inappropriate guilt, eating and/or sleeping problems, excessive tiredness, and lack of concentration that interfere significantly with all facets of daily functioning. Because of its chronic and recurring nature, along with high rates of comorbid disorders and the pronounced risk for mortality due to suicidal behavior and self-harm, depression constitutes a major public health priority (American Psychiatric Association 2013).

One of the signature features of depressive phenomenology is a systematically negative cognitive bias when thinking about oneself, the world, and the future (the cognitive triad) (Beck et al. 1979). This negative thinking style is so pervasive that it sets off a self-destructive downward spiral of low mood and maladaptive behavior, feeding back to negative cognition. Mindfulness holds significant promise in breaking this cycle of depression by safeguarding individuals from this harsh, overly critical cognitive style. Mindfulness training teaches individuals to become more aware of thoughts and feelings yet at the same time to "decenter" from these inner experiences by detaching from them and treating them as "mental events" rather than actual facts (Teasdale et al. 2000). This *decentering* effect soothes the negativity and prevents distorted cognitions from escalating further, impeding the downward direction of the spiral.

What is perhaps most concerning about depression is that it tends to follow an increasingly enduring course. Maintenance antidepressant medication is the

TABLE 6–1. Characteristics of mindfulness-based interventions

Name	Developer (year)	Format	Treatment goals and techniques	Targeted disorders
Mindfulness-Based Stress Reduction (MBSR)	Kabat-Zinn (1990)	8-week intensive program with weekly group meetings lasting 2.5–3 hours	Aims to reduce prolonged periods of stress that are linked to poor physical and mental health outcomes. Techniques: 1) Hatha yoga, 2) sitting meditation, 3) body scans (sustained mindfulness practice in which attention is sequentially directed throughout the body)	Anxiety, depression, (chronic) physical illness
Mindfulness-Based Cognitive Therapy (MBCT)	Segal et al. (2002)	8-week program with weekly group sessions lasting 2–3 hours plus one whole-day session	Aims to interrupt ruminative processes by cultivating decentered awareness to prevent depressive relapse. Techniques: 1) MBSR techniques (i.e., meditation, breathing exercises and stretching), 2) cognitive-behavioral techniques (i.e., linking thoughts with feelings; psychoeducation on the nature of depression and relapse prevention), 3) use of metaphors and poetry	Recurrent depression, bipolar disorder, anxiety disorders, chronic fatigue
Mindfulness-Based Relapse Prevention (MBRP)	Bowen et al. (2011)	8-week program with weekly group sessions lasting 2 hours	Aims to identify and modify deficits in coping skills and self-efficacy. Techniques: 1) focus on the lifestyle balance, 2) relapse management techniques (exercise; reading; meditation, including imagery)	Substance use, depression, eating disorders, schizophrenia, bipolar disorder, erectile dysfunction

TABLE 6–1. Characteristics of mindfulness-based interventions *(continued)*

Name	Developer (year)	Format	Treatment goals and techniques	Targeted disorders
Mindfulness-Based Eating Awareness Training (MB-EAT)	Kristeller and Hallett (1999)	10 core weekly sessions and 2 monthly follow-up sessions	Aims to cultivate mindful attention to and awareness of the eating experience, improve emotion regulation, and change relationship with food. Techniques: 1) emotional eating visualization, 2) breath awareness, 3) body scan practice, 4) healing self-touch, 5) chair yoga	Binge-eating disorder, compulsive overeating and weight management difficulties, type 2 diabetes, bulimia nervosa
Person-Based Cognitive Therapy (PBCT)	Chadwick (2006)	8–12 weekly 90-minute group sessions	Integrates traditional cognitive-behavioral therapy for psychosis and mindfulness practice. Aims to increase acceptance of voice hearing and promote the formation of a more fluid sense of self. Techniques: 1) 10-minute formal mindfulness exercises, 2) reflective group discussion using a guided discovery approach focusing on identifying and altering unhelpful beliefs about voices, negative or maladaptive beliefs about self and others (schemas), and relationship with voices	Psychotic disorders (e.g., schizophrenia, schizoaffective disorder)

first line of treatment for preventing relapse; however, a large percentage of depressed patients find it hard to adhere to antidepressant medications for long periods. Therefore, not surprisingly, relapse rates are as high as 50%–80% (American Psychiatric Association 2013). MBCT (Segal et al. 2002), which combines elements from cognitive therapy for severe depression with intensive training in mindfulness meditation, was developed as an alternative maintenance treatment for patients with a history of recurrent depression. Rather than challenging or changing specific cognitions, as taught in cognitive-behavioral therapy (CBT), MBCT focuses on teaching patients effective ways to relate to depressive thoughts and feelings. First, it cultivates awareness of negative thoughts and feelings at times of potential recurrence of symptoms. Second, it trains patients to relate to their unpleasant thoughts, feelings, and bodily sensations as temporary products of the mind rather than identifying with them or treating them as accurate reflections of reality.

A large number of clinical trials and meta-analyses have established the effectiveness of MBCT as a prophylactic treatment for recurrent major depression (e.g., Khoury et al. 2013; Piet and Hougaard 2011). Evidence also suggests that MBCT may provide significant protection against suicidal recurrent depression (Barnhofer et al. 2015). Interestingly, MBCT may be of more help to patients who are most vulnerable to relapse; although of little benefit in patients with one or two past episodes, MBCT has been found to reduce the risk of relapse or recurrence of depression by 43% compared with treatment as usual or placebo (Piet and Hougaard 2011). Onset of depression at earlier ages and adversity or abuse in childhood are additional treatment moderators that appear to maximize treatment gains of MBCT (Williams et al. 2014).

Growing evidence suggests that MBCT can also be effective for actively depressed and anxious patients in primary care settings, patients with active treatment-resistant depression, and medically ill patients (Piet et al. 2012; Vøllestad et al. 2012). Preliminary evidence supports the clinical utility of MBCT as a treatment adapted for perinatal depression (MBCT-PD; Dimidjian et al. 2016). Another mindfulness intervention showing promising results in the treatment of depression is MBSR, particularly as a treatment for stress and mood symptoms among physically ill patients (Gotink et al. 2015). However, the robustness of this body of research is compromised by several methodological shortcomings, including small sample sizes and absence of a control group, thus warranting further investigation.

The salutary effect of mindfulness training on depression prophylaxis has further been supported by neuroimaging research. Studies investigating long-term effects of mindfulness practice have found that cerebral areas and subcortical structures involved in attentional processes tend to be thicker in subjects who practiced mindfulness than in control subjects (Chiesa and Serretti 2010).

However, the mechanisms underlying depressive symptom reduction with MBIs are not fully known. Putative mechanisms include the development of metacognitive and emotion regulation skills, along with the ability to understand and forestall ruminative cognitive processing, all of which play a pivotal role in the prevention of future depressive episodes.

Anxiety Disorders

Anxiety is a natural response against potentially threatening circumstances, characterized by unpleasant feelings of uneasiness and worry that are often accompanied by restlessness, impaired concentration, and muscular tension. Anxiety disorders, on the other hand, emerge as an exaggerated and out-of-proportion reaction to a perceived threat. Individuals with anxiety disorders experience marked distress, physiological arousal, and fearfulness and tend to engage in excessively avoidant behavior, all of which result in significant interference with daily functioning (American Psychiatric Association 2013).

The theoretical principle of mindfulness practice stands in sharp contrast with the nature of anxiety. Contrary to anxiety, which is characterized by a future-oriented emotional state, mindfulness attends to present experience. Whereas anxiety can lead to a fleeing away from potentially threatening circumstances, mindfulness advocates for an open and accepting attitude in attending to one's own experience. Moreover, through the holistic, mind-body techniques used in mindfulness practice, participants learn to better regulate the physical symptoms of anxiety and to attend to distressing experiences in a more "objective" and detached way.

The most popular and empirically supported stress-management mindfulness program, Kabat-Zinn's (1990) MBSR, incorporates several exercises and topics to make mindfulness more easily accessible to the practitioner. In MBSR, patients are encouraged to mindfully observe and accept anxiety-related thoughts and emotions to witness and attend to unpleasant internal experience by cultivating an open and nonjudgmental stance. In contrast to CBT, the "gold standard" intervention for anxiety disorders, which employs in vivo or imagery exposure to feared stimuli in its core repertoire of strategies for anxiety treatment, MBSR does not implement formal behavioral exposure procedures. However, by promoting an open and nonjudgmental observation of internal states, MBSR does offer an alternative, less direct exposure against experiential avoidance typically observed in anxiety disorders. Additionally, MBSR promotes a more holistic understanding of anxiety and stress, and rather than psychoeducating patients on anxiety symptoms or reappraising and modifying the cognitive content, it focuses more broadly on making the individual focus his or her attention on the moment as well as relate to the current experience in an open and accepting manner.

Evidence from clinical trials and meta-analyses provide support for the effectiveness of MBIs in anxiety disorders. However, only a small fraction of this research derives from randomized controlled designs that compare MBIs with control groups and other active treatments. Overall, MBIs, and MBSR and MBCT in particular, are moderately efficacious for anxiety disorders, and their positive effects are maintained long after treatment (de Vibe et al. 2012; Hofmann et al. 2010; Strauss et al. 2014). The emphasis of MBSR on the continuation of mindfulness practice outside the therapy room following treatment termination may play a pivotal role in helping patients solidify their therapeutic gains. That being said, MBIs are not efficacious for all types of anxiety disorders; one interesting finding is that MBIs may confer more beneficial effects in anxiety disorders with a mixed and heterogeneous clinical picture (Vøllestad et al. 2012).

Trauma and Stress-Related Disorders

Individuals with posttraumatic stress disorder (PTSD) and other trauma-related conditions usually avoid reminders of the trauma and display increased anxiety, emotional arousal, and experiential avoidance (American Psychiatric Association 2013). Mindfulness training involves fostering awareness and acceptance of the present experience in an open, nonjudgmental way. Thus, this training can be greatly beneficial for individuals with trauma-related thoughts or emotions because it may serve as an indirect mechanism of cognitive-affective exposure.

MBIs show promise as interventions for PTSD. Preliminary studies found MBIs to significantly decrease PTSD and depression symptoms, reduce experiential avoidance, and promote emotion regulation (Vujanovic et al. 2016). Nevertheless, the effectiveness of integrating mindfulness-based practices into existing PTSD interventions needs to be further investigated. Evidence deriving from randomized controlled trials is needed to determine the clinical utility of MBIs for PTSD, as well as any possible contraindications, because some concerns have been voiced about the risk of mindfulness-based practices actually causing emotional flooding and retraumatization of certain patients with PTSD.

The mechanisms by which MBIs bring about symptom relief in patients with PTSD remain to be empirically tested. One possible mechanism is that mindfulness eliminates avoidance behaviors, which are well-established contributors to maintaining PTSD symptoms over time. Mindfulness practice encourages participants to bring forth an attitude of curiosity and openness to experience, which often includes difficult traumatic experience (Brown et al. 2007). Moreover, the acquisition of the ability to deal with distressing thoughts or emotions with sustained nonjudgmental attention helps to reduce hypervigilance and emotional numbing. Additionally, a decrease in rumination has been shown to mediate the relationship between beliefs about the trauma and current PTSD symptomatology (Bennett and Wells 2010).

Attention-Deficit/Hyperactivity Disorder

ADHD is characterized by persistent and developmentally inappropriate symptoms of inattention, hyperactivity, and impulsivity that result in significant impairment in major areas of daily functioning (American Psychiatric Association 2013). Individuals with ADHD have marked difficulty organizing tasks and activities, fail to pay close attention to details, and are easily distractible, showing impairments in their ability to sustain their attention to the task at hand; they may also engage in excessive talking or fidgeting and show marked difficulty inhibiting their responses.

Mindfulness simultaneously targets neurocognitive deficits in attention, associated difficulties with inhibition and impulsivity, and secondary symptoms of stress, anxiety, and depression that too often accompany the clinical picture of ADHD. The core element of mindfulness that should benefit patients with ADHD is the self-regulation of attention, a strategy that helps participants to orient to the present moment in a nonjudgmental and accepting way. Participants are initially encouraged to focus on their breathing, a technique geared toward strengthening sustained attention and concentration, and to gradually broaden the focus of their awareness toward monitoring all the experienced mental, emotional, or sensory internal experiences. This technique teaches engagement in emotional states by initiating a mindful way of processing each emotion rather than a mindless one (i.e., avoidance, flooding, or dissociation). In addition, shifting attention to a neutral stimulus (breath or a certain body location) may help the individual detach from harsh emotional states.

Mindfulness training has been implemented for children and adolescents with ADHD as a child-focused intervention, with promising results (Zoogman et al. 2015). Preliminary results from MBI studies show a decrease of ADHD symptoms such as inattention, hyperactive-impulsive behavior, and poor monitoring skills, as well as improvement in social problems and in some secondary internalizing and externalizing symptoms such as symptoms of anxiety, depression, oppositional defiant behavior, and conduct disorder (Mitchell et al. 2015). Equally promising is the evidence from mindfulness programs targeting adult ADHD. Findings from these studies suggest significant pre- to postintervention improvements, which include decreases in inattentive, hyperactive-impulsive, anxious, and depressive symptoms, as well as an increase in emotion regulation, all of which were sustained after a 3-month follow-up (Mitchell et al. 2015).

One prominent way in which mindfulness exerts its positive effects on patients with ADHD is the enhancement of emotion regulation and attentional control, which helps to decrease individuals' mind-wandering when they are faced with multiple, conflicting inputs. Findings from neuroimaging studies suggest that mindfulness meditation engenders neuroplastic changes in brain areas implicated in attentional functioning that is typically impaired in ADHD, such as the anterior cingulate cortex (Hölzel et al. 2011).

Eating Disorders

Eating disorders are characterized by significantly disturbed eating patterns, including compulsive eating or restrictive dieting. Eating disorders are a group of serious disorders, associated with significant distress and functional impairment, high rates of comorbid disorders including anxiety and mood symptoms, substance abuse, and physical impediments, leading to a diminished quality of life. Mindfulness training has been adapted to address a wide range of eating-related issues. The reasoning behind the application of mindfulness as a treatment for eating disorders pertains to the powerful effect of MBIs in promoting awareness of internal experiences, including emotions and physical sensations, with the aim of helping patients learn to regulate their emotions effectively while encouraging the development of self-acceptance, cognitive flexibility, compassion, and forgiveness (Baer et al. 2005; Kristeller and Hallett 1999).

Mindfulness-Based Eating Awareness Training (MB-EAT; Kristeller and Hallett 1999) has been developed to address a broad range of food intake regulation problems, particularly binge-eating disorder. The MB-EAT program is aimed at cultivating nonjudgmental awareness and acceptance of internal experiences and food preferences; it integrates traditional mindfulness and meditation elements of the MBSR module (e.g., breath regulation, sitting meditation) with techniques focused on eating disturbances (e.g., emotional vs. physical hunger triggers, mindful eating). Originally developed for the treatment of eating disorders, MB-EAT has been adapted to target a range of eating-related issues, including type 2 diabetes, and to help individuals with weight management difficulties.

Empirical evidence on MBIs for eating disorders appears to show promising treatment effects, especially for binge-eating disorder and other atypical eating disorders such as compulsive overeating and emotional eating (Katterman et al. 2014; Masuda and Hill 2013). Findings from a three-armed randomized controlled trial by Kristeller and colleagues provide evidence for the efficacy of MB-EAT in reducing symptoms of binge-eating disorder; preliminary results also suggest that MBCT may be efficacious in reducing binge-eating episodes and emotional eating and improving body image (for a review, see Katterman et al. 2014). Further investigation is warranted because these studies were limited by small sample sizes and await replication to determine the comparative and long-term effectiveness of the interventions. Evidence is very limited for MBIs as treatments for anorexia nervosa and bulimia, although blended interventions containing elements of mindfulness practice, such as DBT and ACT, hold promise as treatments for these disorders (Katterman et al. 2014).

Substance-Related and Addictive Disorders

Substance-related disorders are mainly characterized by a pattern of prolonged, excessive use of a medication, non–medically indicated drug, or toxin, which leads to significant functional impairment, whereas addictive disorders are activities and behavioral patterns that have become uncontrollable (American Psychiatric Association 2013). Substance-related and addictive disorders are linked to high mortality rates, thus indicating an urgent need for a treatment that focuses on relapse prevention.

The theoretical principles of mindfulness hold invaluable clinical utility for the treatment of addictive disorders. The central premise of mindfulness is to cultivate an intentional and accepting switch of one's attention toward present-moment experience, which is in sharp contrast to cognitive and affective states commonly observed in substance use disorders. Individuals struggling with substance misuse are characterized by considerable experiential avoidance, often running on "autopilot" to block painful and distressing stimuli from entering into their full awareness. This escapist tendency serves the important function of distancing these individuals from unpleasant sensations that would potentially lead to craving and ultimately relapse; however, this tendency does not appear to be a feasible long-term strategy, as is corroborated by the strikingly high rates of relapse among this clinical population. Mindfulness offers an alternative way of attending to these highly distressing and unwanted internal states. Capitalizing on the healing power of meditative practice, participants learn to "surf the urge" rather than respond to cravings in either a suppressing or a reactive manner.

Mounting evidence supports the clinical utility of MBIs in treating substance use disorders. More specifically, mindfulness training has been linked to significant reductions in consumption of substances, including alcohol, cocaine, amphetamines, marijuana, tobacco, and opiates (Chiesa et al. 2014; Zgierska et al. 2009). The treatment that is most supported by research thus far is Mindfulness-Based Relapse Prevention (MBRP; Bowen et al. 2011), a mindfulness-based aftercare package that incorporates MBSR and MBCT strategies within a relapse prevention framework. MBRP trains participants to recognize "red flags" and early signs for relapse and cultivates awareness of cravings as well as internal affective states related to substance using, thereby helping them to respond more adaptively over time.

Psychosis

Schizophrenia spectrum disorders are a group of severe mental disorders characterized by hallucinations, delusions, and cognitive and behavioral disorganization, as well as varying levels of motivational impairment, cognitive deficits, and poor interpersonal functioning (American Psychiatric Association 2013). Although treatment with antipsychotic drugs reduces the hallucinations and delusions of schizophrenia, this treatment has little impact on negative symptoms, medication compliance, and general well-being. Psychosocial interventions are tremendously valuable adjuncts to medication in terms of improving the health and social outcomes of people living with schizophrenia. Mindfulness in particular can be a valuable tool in promoting psychological well-being by increasing patients' tolerance of disturbing internal stimuli and normalizing their psychotic sensory experiences through various guided meditation techniques.

Concerns have been raised regarding the clinical utility and safe implementation of MBIs for people with such severe symptomatology, on the basis that early studies revealed poor treatment outcomes for patients with psychosis. Although these concerns have some merit, these early studies were largely uncontrolled and employed nonmanualized and nonadapted mindfulness practices for patients with psychosis (Chadwick 2014). Indeed, standard meditation practices may be too overwhelming for individuals who respond to internal stimuli in the context of a psychotic disorder. Therefore, certain adaptations in meditation practice are necessary to render the treatment feasible, tolerable, and safe for this population.

One such mindfulness treatment is Person-Based Cognitive Therapy (PBCT; Chadwick 2006). PBCT integrates traditional cognitive therapy for psychosis with mindfulness- and acceptance-based practices and aims at reducing distress triggered by hearing voices. Mindfulness practice in PBCT has undergone several alterations, such as avoiding long silences and making the mindfulness practice much shorter, structured, and guided (Chadwick 2006; see Table 6.1).

Contemporary evidence from meta-analyses of evidence-based mindfulness packages shows that MBIs are moderately effective in alleviating negative symptoms and can be useful adjuncts to pharmacotherapy (Khoury et al. 2013). However, these findings are limited by the small number of MBI randomized, controlled studies in this patient population.

Toward Personalized Mindfulness-Based Treatment

Growing evidence shows that MBIs are effective for a variety of mental disorders and populations. However, little is known about the specific mechanisms by which mindfulness exerts its beneficial effects. Despite the proliferation of research investigating the efficacy of MBIs on mental health disorders, few research studies have attempted to study the mechanisms of therapeutic change in mindfulness training programs; in other words, research on mechanisms has not caught up yet with efficacy trials.

Similarly, there is a striking dearth of research exploring treatment moderators—namely, factors that would help clarify for what subgroup of patients mindfulness may be particularly effective—and, relatedly, the circumstances under which mindfulness might be less helpful, or even harmful, compared with other treatments. Preliminary evidence suggests that the effectiveness of MBIs is influenced by clinical characteristics, including the number of previous depressive episodes experienced by a patient with recurrent depression, the baseline severity of depression, and the level of anxiety sensitivity, along with personality traits (de Vibe et al. 2015). The effectiveness of MBIs is also influenced by treatment characteristics, such as the duration of the intervention and the implementation of homework practice, and therapist characteristics, such as the mindfulness training of the therapist, although research on these factors has yielded contradictory findings (Khoury et al. 2013).

Mindfulness is a promising therapeutic tool in the treatment of a wide range of psychopathology, but it is by no means a panacea that cures all ailments. Rather, it is a complex and multidimensional therapeutic intervention targeting different problem areas. As such, patients are more likely to benefit from mindfulness strategies that target their particular difficulties and address their unique treatment needs. For example, disorders that primarily involve attentional impairment, such as ADHD, may require that the attentional aspect of mindfulness training be emphasized more. On the other hand, for disorders with the symptom of excessive guilt, such as eating disorders or depression, treatment may be more efficient if it focuses primarily on acceptance and self-compassion.

In this section, we briefly present psychological mechanisms that either remain theoretical or have been empirically assessed and describe some of the criteria to be considered as mediators. A solid understanding of how these mechanisms work and how the specific components of mindfulness are linked to positive outcomes is crucial for practitioners to successfully apply the problem formulation approach and leverage their therapeutic benefits.

Factors of Therapeutic Change

It has been suggested that MBIs include three main factors that contribute significantly in the process of improving self-regulation: 1) enhanced control of attention, 2) efficient emotion regulation, and 3) insightful self-awareness (Hölzel et al. 2011; Tang et al. 2015). Several theoretical models, or mechanisms, have been proposed to describe the underlying processes by which MBIs bring about physical and psychological changes (Table 6–2). Each of these mechanisms offers different hypothesized mechanisms of change. We further explore the specific processes underlying the three main factors.

Control of Attention

One well-documented mechanism by which mindfulness practice confers its beneficial effects is through improving participants' ability to regulate and con-

TABLE 6–2. Factors of therapeutic change

Factor	Description	Techniques	Targeted disorders	Brain-related areas
Attentional control	Multifaceted attentional process consisting of 1) alerting, 2) orienting, and 3) conflict monitoring	Yoga, breath regulation, focused attention meditation	Attention-deficit/hyperactivity disorder, depressive disorders	Right frontal and parietal cortex and thalamus, anterior cingulate cortex, superior colliculus, prefrontal cortex, basal ganglia (Malinowski 2013; Tang et al. 2015)
Emotion regulation: reappraisal and acceptance	Altering emotional content by adopting an open, curious, and accepting attitude	Yoga, sitting meditation, body scans	Stress and pain-related symptoms	Dorsal prefrontal cortex (Tang et al. 2015)
Emotion regulation: exposure	Engaging with distressing stimuli to overcome experiential avoidance	Breathing exercises, acceptance-based techniques, decentering, nonevaluative awareness	Depressive disorders, anxiety disorders, obsessive-compulsive disorders, substance use disorders	Ventromedial prefrontal cortex, hippocampus, amygdala (medial/superior frontal region), anterior cingulate cortex (Tang et al. 2015)
Self-awareness: meta-awareness	Cognitive set in which negative thoughts and feelings are experienced as mental events rather than as the self	Yoga, meditation, body scans	Recurrent major depressive disorder/depressive symptoms relapse	Right rostrolateral prefrontal cortex, contralateral prefrontal cortex, visual cortex (Fleming et al. 2012)

TABLE 6–2.   Factors of therapeutic change *(continued)*

Factor	Description	Techniques	Targeted disorders	Brain-related areas
Self-awareness: self-compassion	Process of empathizing with one's own suffering and having the desire to treat self with understanding and concern	Diffusion, values authorship, willingness in compassionate exposure, nonjudgmental present-moment attention	Depressive relapse; eating, anxiety, and bipolar disorders; substance use (e.g., smoking cessation)	Insula; amygdala, right temporoparietal junction, right posterior superior temporal sulcus (circuits implicated in empathy) (Lutz et al. 2008)
Self-awareness: values clarification	Process whereby an individual identifies his or her values, goals, meaning, and purpose in life and makes decisions congruent with these values	Mindfulness, meditation, homework exercises	Depression, suicidality, anxiety	No published data on brain-related areas

trol their attention (Bishop et al. 2004). The rather complex mechanism of attentional control implicates various neurobiologically distinct attention subsystems: 1) alerting, or the ability to maintain a vigilant and receptive state with respect to a wide range of potential stimuli; 2) orienting, or the ability to direct and sustain attention toward a subset of possible inputs in the present moment; and 3) conflict monitoring, or the ability to prioritize among competing inputs and distracting tasks and to switch attention back and forth whenever it wanders (Anderson et al. 2007; Jha et al. 2007). The mechanism of attentional control plays a pivotal role in the treatment of various disorders, including depression and ADHD, among others (Chambers et al. 2008), and has been found to exert an antiruminative effect on cognitive-emotional processes. Findings from experimental studies using various neuropsychological tasks provide evidence for the positive impact of mindfulness training in attentional control (Jha et al. 2007).

Emotion Regulation

Improved emotion regulation results from learning strategies to help control what kind of emotions arise and when, how long they last, and how they are experienced and conveyed. Emotion regulation is a complex and multifaceted process, involving a variety of more targeted regulatory mechanisms. The two with the most supporting evidence are 1) reappraisal and acceptance and 2) exposure.

Acceptance is an emotion-regulation mechanism that entails *reappraising* the emotional content of a particular experience by adopting an open, curious, and accepting attitude. It derives from loving-kindness Buddhist practice and is used to gradually impede the development of mental states that are linked to aversion. Essentially, when practicing mindfulness, individuals are encouraged to attend to their present experience in a nonjudgmental way, whatever the content of these thoughts, sensations, or feelings is. Moreover, at times when their mind starts wandering, they are instructed to "observe" their mind becoming distracted and gently bring it back to the here and now, without any negative labeling or judgment. Acceptance, therefore, is a powerful mechanism that shields individuals against aversive emotional states while equipping them with essential emotional self-regulation skills.

Another process hypothesized to take place during mindfulness practice is exposure. By intentionally attending to experiences in a nonjudgmental and accepting manner, an individual may undergo a process of desensitization equivalent to traditional exposure elements implemented in behavioral treatments. Mindfulness participants are encouraged to sit with and experience distressing bodily sensations, thoughts, or emotions as passing mental events that are not to be avoided or suppressed; this alone allows for habituation to and a reduction of the level of distress. Thus, meditative practices in mindfulness facilitate the process of facing aversive stimuli in an indirect and "observing" manner rather than being directly exposed. This is further supported by evidence showing that practicing mindfulness leads to an increase in behavioral activation and functional status along with a decrease in experiential avoidance (Kearney et al. 2012).

Self-Awareness

According to Buddhist philosophy, the identification of the self as a static entity is linked to significant distress. Mindfulness practice is suggested to promote the dissociation from identification with the self as a static entity as well as to instill the quality of experience within the identification process.

An important aspect of self-awareness is *meta-awareness*, defined as the ability to reperceive or to decenter from one's thoughts and emotions and to view them as passing mental events rather than to identify with them or to believe that the thoughts are accurate representations of reality (Teasdale 1999). Increased meta-awareness has been hypothesized to lead to reductions in rumination, a process of repetitive negative thinking that has been considered a transdiagnostic risk factor for a series of mental disorders (Ehring and Watkins 2008). Preliminary evidence suggests that MBIs are linked to an increase in meta-awareness and a decrease in rumination (Bishop et al. 2004). The increased levels of metacognitive awareness, or decentering, may in turn predict better clinical outcomes, such as lower rates of depressive relapses (Fresco et al. 2007; Teasdale et al. 2002).

Another important aspect of self-awareness is *self-compassion*, which entails three major components (Neff 2003): 1) self-kindness—the ability to be kind and accepting toward one's shortcomings and vulnerabilities, rather than being harshly disapproving of them; 2) common humanity—the capacity to adopt a humanistic stance toward one's experiences rather than treating them as separating and isolating; and 3) mindfulness—a capacity to relate to painful or distressing thoughts and feelings in a balanced and decentered manner, rather than overidentifying with them. Self-compassion is closely related to acceptance.

Another mechanism that takes place during mindfulness is clarification of values (Shapiro et al. 2006). Attending to present experience with curiosity and nonjudgmental attitude helps individuals explore and clarify their values and, consequently, harmonize their behavior with these core values. Preliminary evidence has demonstrated that values clarification partially mediates the relationship between mindfulness training and decreased psychological distress (Carmody et al. 2009).

Problem Formulation Approach

Case Example

Jenna is a 23-year-old single woman who currently works part time at a retail store and lives with her parents. She graduated from college 1 year ago and has struggled to secure full-time employment. She reports that as her financial situation worsened, she became more and more worried and soon began to experience panic attacks when she was traveling to job interviews. She describes that prior to an attack, she often has thoughts such as "I am going to mess up this interview" and "I am worthless" and feels significant bodily tension. During an attack, she reports thinking that she is going to die because she notices that her heart is beating rapidly and her breathing is shallow. She has had these attacks now for 3 months and currently avoids job interviews for fear of having another attack.

Jenna's panic is maintained through her avoidance of situations that she currently labels as dangerous (i.e., going to a job interview). She needs a structured mindfulness program so that she can learn to notice and tolerate her thoughts, feelings, and bodily sensations as she "sits" with these uncomfortable experiences in the therapy room. Over time, she can identify less with these thoughts, feelings, and bodily sensations and through this exposure recalibrate the danger level of these situations. Perhaps she will even come to accept that a certain level of anxiety might be part of her physiological/psychological makeup and simply learn to regard the anxiety as part of her individual experience of the world.

Primary Mechanisms of Change and Treatment Plan

In Jenna's case, metacognitive awareness, exposure, and acceptance are considered the primary mechanisms through which mindfulness can bring about changes in her treatment outcome. Hence, the treatment plan will be formed as follows:

1. **Treatment buy-in:** The clinician introduces the ideas of mindfulness to Jenna in session. Jenna agrees with the rationale that by increasing her ability to stay with her experience nonjudgmentally, her panic symptoms will decrease.
2. **Daily practice:** Jenna begins a daily mindfulness practice. She first practices a short breathing meditation and body scan in session with her clinician and then begins to practice these techniques daily at home. She also begins to bring mindfulness informally into her daily life, noticing her experience nonjudgmentally at various moments throughout her day and performing daily tasks (e.g., brushing her teeth) with mindfulness.
3. **Practice of mindfulness during a panic attack:** As her personal mindfulness practice grows more solid, Jenna then begins to practice mindfulness when confronted with an anxiety-producing situation. First, she practices this with her clinician in session through recalling an experience that brought on a panic attack. Next, she begins to employ mindfulness while she is experiencing a panic attack. Specifically, she consciously and continually brings her awareness to certain experiential anchors: the quality of her

breath (e.g., whether it is fast or slow, shallow or deep), bodily sensations (e.g., tension in shoulders), thoughts (e.g., "I'm going to die"), and emotions (e.g., fear). She then processes her experience of the attack in her next therapy session. Through this inquiry Jenna becomes better at identifying when she is about to experience a panic attack; at recognizing her habitual thoughts, feelings, and bodily sensation during a panic attack; and at developing confidence in her ability to live through the experience of panic. Over time, she becomes able to remain curious about her experience as it is occurring and to remind herself that she is experiencing a panic attack and not a life-threatening situation.

Conclusion and Future Directions

Overall, evidence suggests that MBIs have positive effects for patients with a variety of psychiatric disorders. For example, MBSR and MBCT have significant antidepressant and antianxiety effects and decrease overall psychological distress. However, research is still in its infancy in terms of understanding the psychological and neurobiological effects of these practices. Further mediator- and moderator-based studies are needed to theorize the pathways through which MBIs decrease psychopathology and what particular populations will benefit (Dimidjian and Segal 2015). To date, there is a paucity of high-quality studies (randomized controlled trials) to establish an empirically solid basis for MBIs to leverage their clinical utility. It seems likely that the widespread benefits of mindfulness practice shown in currently available studies may be at least partially explained by its effects on transdiagnostic processes that appear to cut across a series of mental disorders. In addition, because of its nature, mindfulness might be helpful in targeting the chronic and recurring patterns of mental illness, and by virtue of being "client centered," MBIs have the potential for high levels of acceptability compared with traditional, symptom-focused treatment approaches.

Despite the rapid increase of research on the effectiveness of MBIs, critical issues still need to be addressed. The apparent simplicity of MBIs presents the risk that the techniques may be misunderstood, oversimplified, or indiscriminately applied. The developers behind both MBSR and MBCT highlight that it is imperative for the interventions to be delivered by instructors with adequate theoretical knowledge and practical experience. It has been postulated that part of the heterogeneity of treatment outcomes observed in meta-analyses could be attributable to differences in the level of clinical training and experience among instructors. Therefore, future studies need to focus particularly on optimizing adherence rates to mindfulness practice.

Finally, additional empirical attention needs to be given to specific factors that may predict attenuated therapeutic benefits or even harm. An interesting ongoing discussion among experts focuses on the extent to which mindfulness may be counterindicated for acute and destabilizing conditions, such as acute symptoms of PTSD, floridly psychotic states, and active substance use disorders. Especially with regard to trauma, there is some hesitation in implementing meditative techniques; they may have an iatrogenic effect, causing severe dissociative phenomena or flooding the individual with traumatic material.

Key Points for Further Study and Reflection

- Mindfulness-based interventions (MBIs) are considerably heterogeneous (see Table 6–1).
- Mounting evidence supports the clinical utility of MBIs across a wide range of mental disorders. MBIs for depression and anxiety are thus far the most empirically supported interventions.
- MBIs may be more effective if tailored on the basis of specific symptomatology and underlying mechanisms.
- It has been suggested that MBIs include three main components that contribute significantly to the process of improving self-regulation: 1) enhanced control of attention, 2) efficient emotion regulation, and 3) insightful self-awareness.
- The specific mechanisms of therapeutic change that underlie these main components include, among others, acceptance, exposure, meta-awareness, and self-compassion (see Table 6–2).
- The apparent simplicity of MBIs presents the risk that the techniques may be misunderstood, oversimplified, or indiscriminately applied.

References

American Psychiatric Association: Diagnostic and Statistical Manual of Mental Disorders, 5th Edition. Arlington, VA, American Psychiatric Association, 2013

Anderson ND, Lau MA, Segal ZV, Bishop SR: Mindfulness-based stress reduction and attentional control. Clin Psychol Psychother 14(6):449–463, 2007

Baer RA, Fischer S, Huss DB: Mindfulness and acceptance in the treatment of disordered eating. J Ration-Emot Cogn-Behav Ther 23(4):281–300, 2005

Barnhofer T, Crane C, Brennan K, et al: Mindfulness-based cognitive therapy (MBCT) reduces the association between depressive symptoms and suicidal cognitions in patients with a history of suicidal depression. J Consult Clin Psychol 83(6):1013–1020, 2015 26302249

Beck AT, Rush AJ, Shaw BF, Emery G. Cognitive Therapy of Depression. New York, Guilford, 1979

Bennett H, Wells A: Metacognition, memory disorganization and rumination in post-traumatic stress symptoms. J Anxiety Disord 24(3):318–325, 2010 20144524

Bishop SR, Lau M, Shapiro S, et al: Mindfulness: a proposed operational definition. Clin Psychol Sci Pract 11(3):230–241, 2004

Bowen S, Chawla N, Marlatt GA: Mindfulness-Based Relapse Prevention for Addictive Behaviors: A Clinician's Guide. New York, Guilford, 2011

Brown KW, Ryan RM, Creswell JD: Mindfulness: theoretical foundations and evidence for its salutary effects. Psychol Inq 18(4):211–237, 2007

Carmody J, Baer RA, Lykins ELB, Olendzki N: An empirical study of the mechanisms of mindfulness in a mindfulness-based stress reduction program. J Clin Psychol 65(6):613–626, 2009 19267330

Chadwick P: Person-Based Cognitive Therapy for Distressing Psychosis. Chichester, UK, Wiley, 2006

Chadwick P: Mindfulness for psychosis. Br J Psychiatry 204(5):333–334, 2014 24785766

Chambers R, Lo BCY, Allen NB: The impact of intensive mindfulness training on attentional control, cognitive style, and affect. Cognit Ther Res 32(3):303–322, 2008

Chiesa A, Serretti A: A systematic review of neurobiological and clinical features of mindfulness meditations. Psychol Med 40(8):1239–1252, 2010 19941676

Chiesa A, Serretti A: Are mindfulness-based interventions effective for substance use disorders? A systematic review of the evidence. Subst Use Misuse 49(5):492–512, 2014 23461667

de Vibe M, Bjørndal A, Tipton E, et al: Mindfulness based stress reduction (MBSR) for improving health, quality of life, and social functioning in adults. Campbell Syst Rev 127: 2012

de Vibe M, Solhaug I, Tyssen R, et al: Does personality moderate the effects of mindfulness training for medical and psychology students? Mindfulness (NY) 6(2):281–289, 2015 25798208

Dimidjian S, Segal ZV: Prospects for a clinical science of mindfulness-based intervention. Am Psychol 70(7):593–620, 2015 26436311

Dimidjian S, Goodman SH, Felder JN, et al: Staying well during pregnancy and the postpartum: a pilot randomized trial of mindfulness-based cognitive therapy for the prevention of depressive relapse/recurrence. J Consult Clin Psychol 84(2):134–145, 2016 26654212

Ehring T, Watkins ER: Repetitive negative thinking as a transdiagnostic process. Int J Cogn Ther 1(3):192–205, 2008

Fleming SM, Huijgen J, Dolan RJ: Prefrontal contributions to metacognition in perceptual decision making. J Neurosci 32(18):6117–6125, 2012 22553018

Fresco DM, Segal ZV, Buis T, Kennedy S: Relationship of posttreatment decentering and cognitive reactivity to relapse in major depression. J Consult Clin Psychol 75(3):447–455, 2007 17563161

Gotink RA, Chu P, Busschbach JJV, et al: Standardised mindfulness-based interventions in healthcare: an overview of systematic reviews and meta-analyses of RCTs. PLoS One 10(4):e0124344, 2015 25881019

Hofmann SG, Sawyer AT, Witt AA, Oh D: The effect of mindfulness-based therapy on anxiety and depression: a meta-analytic review. J Consult Clin Psychol 78(2):169–183, 2010 20350028

Hölzel BK, Lazar SW, Gard T, et al: How does mindfulness meditation work? Proposing mechanisms of action from a conceptual and neural perspective. Perspect Psychol Sci 6(6):537–559, 2011 26168376

Jha AP, Krompinger J, Baime MJ: Mindfulness training modifies subsystems of attention. Cogn Affect Behav Neurosci 7(2):109–119, 2007 17672382

Kabat-Zinn J: Full Catastrophe Living: Using the Wisdom of Your Body and Mind to Face Stress, Pain, and Illness. New York, Bantam Books, 1990

Katterman SN, Kleinman BM, Hood MM, et al: Mindfulness meditation as an intervention for binge eating, emotional eating, and weight loss: a systematic review. Eat Behav 15(2):197–204, 2014 24854804

Kearney DJ, McDermott K, Malte C, et al: Association of participation in a mindfulness program with measures of PTSD, depression and quality of life in a veteran sample. J Clin Psychol 68(1):101–116, 2012 22125187

Khoury B, Lecomte T, Gaudiano BA, Paquin K: Mindfulness interventions for psychosis: a meta-analysis. Schizophr Res 150(1):176–184, 2013 23954146

Kristeller JL, Hallett CB: An exploratory study of a meditation-based intervention for binge eating disorder. J Health Psychol 4(3):357–363, 1999 22021603

Lutz A, Brefczynski-Lewis J, Johnstone T, Davidson RJ: Regulation of the neural circuitry of emotion by compassion meditation: effects of meditative expertise. PLoS One 3(3):e1897, 2008 18365029

Malinowski P: Neural mechanisms of attentional control in mindfulness meditation. Front Neurosci Feb 4;7·8, 2013 23382709

Masuda A, Hill ML: Mindfulness as therapy for disordered eating: a systematic review. Neuropsychiatry (London) 3:433–447, 2013

Mitchell JT, Zylowska L, Kollins SH: Mindfulness meditation training for attention-deficit/hyperactivity disorder in adulthood: current empirical support, treatment overview, and future directions. Cognit Behav Pract 22(2):172–191, 2015 25908900

Neff K: Self-compassion : an alternative conceptualization of a healthy attitude toward oneself. Self Ident 2:85–101, 2003

Piet J, Hougaard E: The effect of mindfulness-based cognitive therapy for prevention of relapse in recurrent major depressive disorder: a systematic review and meta-analysis. Clin Psychol Rev 31(6):1032–1040, 2011 21802618

Piet J, Würtzen H, Zachariae R: The effect of mindfulness-based therapy on symptoms of anxiety and depression in adult cancer patients and survivors: a systematic review and meta-analysis. J Consult Clin Psychol 80(6):1007–1020, 2012 22563637

Segal Z, Williams M, Teasdale J: Mindfulness-Based Cognitive Therapy for Depression: A New Approach to Preventing Relapse. New York, Guilford, 2002

Shapiro SL, Carlson LE, Astin JA, Freedman B: Mechanisms of mindfulness. J Clin Psychol 62(3):373–386, 2006 16385481

Strauss C, Cavanagh K, Oliver A, Pettman D: Mindfulness-based interventions for people diagnosed with a current episode of an anxiety or depressive disorder: a meta-analysis of randomised controlled trials. PLoS One 9(4):e96110, 2014 24763812

Tang Y-Y, Hölzel BK, Posner MI: The neuroscience of mindfulness meditation. Nat Rev Neurosci 16(4):213–225, 2015 25783612

Teasdale JD: Emotional processing, three modes of mind and the prevention of relapse in depression. Behav Res Ther 37(Suppl 1):S53–S77, 1999 10402696

Teasdale JD, Segal ZV, Williams JM, et al: Prevention of relapse/recurrence in major depression by mindfulness-based cognitive therapy. J Consult Clin Psychol 68(4):615–623, 2000 10965637

Teasdale JD, Moore RG, Hayhurst H, et al: Metacognitive awareness and prevention of relapse in depression: empirical evidence. J Consult Clin Psychol 70(2):275–287, 2002 11952186

Vøllestad J, Nielsen MB, Nielsen GH: Mindfulness- and acceptance-based interventions for anxiety disorders: a systematic review and meta-analysis. Br J Clin Psychol 51(3):239–260, 2012 22803933

Vujanovic AA, Niles BL, Abrams JL: Mindfulness and meditation in the conceptualization and treatment of posttraumatic stress disorder, in Mindfulness and Buddhist-Derived Approaches in Mental Health and Addiction. Edited by Shonin E, Gordon W Van, Griffiths MD. New York, Springer, 2016, pp 225–245

Williams JMG, Crane C, Barnhofer T, et al: Mindfulness-based cognitive therapy for preventing relapse in recurrent depression: a randomized dismantling trial. J Consult Clin Psychol 82(2):275–286, 2014 24294837

Zgierska A, Rabago D, Chawla N, et al: Mindfulness meditation for substance use disorders: a systematic review. Subst Abus 30(4):266–294, 2009 19904664

Zoogman S, Goldberg SB, Hoyt WT, Miller L: Mindfulness interventions with youth: a meta-analysis. Mindfulness 6(2):290–302, 2015

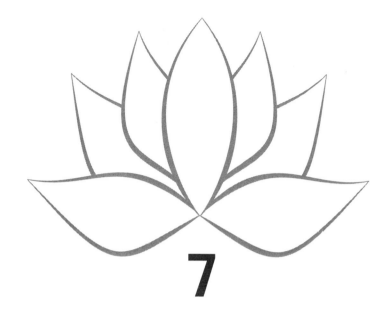

7

Finding Wellness Through Mindfulness and Meditation

The Growing Fields of Positive Psychology and Psychiatry

Cory Muscara, MAPP
Abigail Mengers, MAPP
Alan Schlechter, M.D.

If we take man as he is, we make him worse, but if we take man as he should be, we make him capable of becoming what he can be.

Johann Wolfgang von Goethe

THERE IS A GLOBAL SHIFT taking place in our culture, one inclined toward questioning and understanding what happiness, well-being, and the good life entail. For evidence of this shift, one need only consider that organizations such as Zappos now employ a "chief happiness officer" responsible for the well-being of their employees ("Tony Hsieh, Chief Happiness Officer" 2015); countries such as Bhutan replaced the gross domestic product with a gross national happiness index (Kelly 2012); and organizations such as Mindful Schools have trained thousands of teachers across the country to bring mindfulness meditation into school classrooms (Mindful Schools 2016). All of these actions have emerged in the wake of recent scientific research supporting the many benefits of well-being.

Although well-being has been a subject of interest and inquiry for millennia—from the Buddha's quest for enlightenment more than 2,600 years ago to the articulations of *eudaimonia* in ancient Greece—only recently has this topic gained any traction within the scientific community. This is due in large part to the founding of positive psychology, a field that aims to understand well-being and human flourishing through science.

When Martin Seligman became president of the American Psychological Association in 1998, he stated that the field of psychology of the late twentieth century had not played a large enough role in making the lives of all people better (Seligman 1999). Prior to World War II, the mission of psychology was to cure mental illness, help all people lead more productive and fulfilling lives, and identify and nurture high talent in people. In his presidential address, Seligman argued that after the war, psychology had neglected the latter two intentions of this mission. At the time of his address, for every 17 research articles devoted to negatively oriented emotions, there was only one article on positively oriented emotions. Seligman stated the need for a science that also sought to understand the most positive qualities of individuals—that is, what is "best" in people—and ways to cultivate these qualities.

From that point on, there has been a surge in research and public interest on the topic of well-being, sparking what Pawelski and Moores (2013) refer to as the eudaimonic turn. The *eudaimonic turn* refers to a widespread shift in society in which scholars across a large number of disciplines are focusing less on the causal elements of what is going *wrong* in people, organizations, and communities and more on what is going *right*.

But what does it mean for things to be going right, especially with something as big and complex as a person's life? This is the focus of much scholarship in positive psychology, as numerous conceptions have been offered for what comprises well-being and/or what constitutes the good life. As people go about building their lives, what are the objectives they should be working toward? What are the standards by which they should measure themselves when they want to know how things are going?

For well-being to be measurable, it must be operationalized. To capture the nuances of such a construct, Seligman (2011) created a theory of well-being that can be neatly encapsulated in the acronym PERMA, which stands for **P**ositive emotions, **E**ngagement, (positive) **R**elationships, **M**eaning/purpose, and **A**ccomplishment/achievement. Seligman selected these five elements on the basis of three criteria: First, and perhaps most obviously, each element must individually contribute to well-being. Second, given a choice, people must seek out each of these elements for its own sake and not merely as a means to a different end. Third, each of these elements can be separately measured, subjectively and/or objectively. When people have high scores on each element of PERMA, they are flourishing.

Mindfulness is a key resource to support people who aim to build a flourishing life that includes PERMA. Historically, mindfulness has been associated with the practice of Buddhist meditation, and to this day it remains a central tenet in the Buddhist pursuit of enlightenment. Within the last few decades, however, mindfulness has become recognized as a secular practice to strengthen the mind and body, and it is widely used as an evidence-based modality for improving health, performance, and well-being in settings such as health care, schools, and businesses (Pinsker 2015).

Cultivating and understanding the domain of mind called "awareness" is a fundamental pillar of mindfulness practice. Awareness is the human capacity to know one's experience as it is happening. In psychology, this is sometimes referred to as *metacognition*—awareness and understanding of one's own thought processes. Other forms of awareness are also included in this category, such as *interoception*—the felt sense of one's physiological state—and *proprioception*—the felt sense of the body moving through space.

Have you ever noticed that you can be aware of your thoughts without *thinking* about your thoughts? If not, try it. This awareness is mindfulness—awareness not of the thought itself, or even the absence of thought, but awareness simply that the thought is there. By being mindful in this way, people can purposefully reflect on their experience or take an intentional pause during stressful moments, thus enabling them to *respond* to thoughts and emotions instead of reacting in an unskillful way. The value of being mindful is expressed in Viktor Frankl's (1946/1985) book *Man's Search for Meaning*, in which he describes that the space between stimulus and response is where we have power to choose our response in each moment, thus leading to our growth and freedom. In this space, skillful responses can take place in relation to both positive and negative experiences; that is, we can both enhance the positive and ameliorate the negative.

Additionally, awareness can serve as a top-down or a bottom-up approach. According to a bottom-up approach, awareness provides the soil from which choice and action around well-being can sprout because it is only through awareness that we can make an intentional choice in response to our perceived situation. According to a top-down approach, awareness monitors our experiential state, illuminating cues about current levels of well-being. With these cues, we are able to use other mental processes to negotiate the next step. The more aware we are, the more we know, and thus the better we can respond skillfully to the situation at hand.

When we move through life on automatic pilot, unconscious of our experience, we typically *react* to whatever is presented to us—be it thoughts, emotions, or difficult people—without recognizing the ability to *choose* our response in those moments (Kabat-Zinn 1990). The ability to respond separates our experience from an animal-like reactivity to biological and social cues. In this chapter we focus on how we can enhance the five pillars of PERMA by learning to inhabit this space between stimulus and response through the cultivation of mindful awareness.

Positive Emotions

Positive emotions include not just happiness but also joy, gratitude, serenity, interest, hope, pride, amusement, inspiration, awe, and love, among others (Fredrickson 2009). Mindfulness and meditation can provide a pathway to greater well-being by increasing positive emotions, both directly and indirectly. Practitioners of meditation often report the development of pleasant feelings while meditating, and over time, there may be trait benefits from consistent practice, which can elicit the development of greater serenity and calm. Certain types of meditation, such as loving-kindness meditation (LKM), are even dedicated to encouraging practitioners to extend the feelings of love and connection to those around them. Finally, by developing heightened attention and attunement to novelty through mindfulness, practitioners can experience increased levels of positive emotions in activities outside of and unrelated to meditation, such as eating, parenting, and working.

The study of positive emotions has been a cornerstone of the positive psychology movement. On the surface, it seems rather simple: positive emotions feel good. Because of this, it makes sense that a field seeking to understand and improve well-being would want to know more about something that seems to indicate a basic level of flourishing in the present moment. However, could positive emotions reach beyond their temporary nature and actually increase well-being in the future, instead of just signaling it in the here and now? This is what Barbara Fredrickson (2001) sought to uncover in the development of her broaden-and-build theory of positive emotions.

When Fredrickson (2001) posited the broaden-and-build theory, much more was known about the mechanisms and evolutionary utility of negative emotions than those of positive emotions. For instance, research had shown that when experiencing fear, disgust, or anger, people tend to exhibit certain thoughts, behaviors, and physiological responses that would enable them to confront or distance themselves from the instigating situation. These responses, known as specific action tendencies, were not apparent during the experience of positive emotions. In fact, whereas negative emotions constricted people's courses of action, positive emotions seemed to do the opposite, making it unclear what purpose they served at all.

Fredrickson attempted to show through her theory that positive emotions were adaptive and beneficial to humans, precisely because they allowed people to broaden their perspectives and entertain a wider array of ideas and behaviors. She demonstrated that by broadening people's thought-action repertoires, positive emotions helped people to increase enduring personal resources. For instance, positive emotions can increase intellectual resources by inspiring new ideas through sparking creativity and the formulation of future goals, increase physical resources by causing people to want to explore and engage in playful behavior, and increase social resources by instilling in people the desire to reach out to others in an effort to share the experience of positive emotions, thereby developing relationships through bonding (Fredrickson 2001). Research has also shown that positive emotions undo the potential physically deleterious cardiovascular effects of negative emotions while also building psychological resilience (Fredrickson et al. 2000). Positive emotions have the potential to expand people's mindsets and lead them to accumulate new resources that they can draw on in the future. In this way, the benefits of positive emotions extend beyond the present moment and contribute to a person's increased well-being at a later time.

In two experiments meant to test the broaden-and-build theory, Fredrickson and colleagues used LKM to induce positive emotions in participants (Fredrickson et al. 2008; Kok et al. 2013). Although similar to other types of meditation centered around mindfulness, LKM focuses not just on awareness and attention to the present moment but also on cultivating feelings of love and compassion for the self and then extending those feelings outward to family, friends, and eventually strangers (Fredrickson et al. 2008). LKM was also chosen as a catalyst for positive emotions in these studies because it incorporates emotions into its practice and requires active attention.

In the first study, adults in a workplace sample were randomly assigned either to a 7-week LKM workshop or to a waitlist control group (Fredrickson et al. 2008). The results showed that those participants practicing LKM had increased positive emotion during the meditation sessions and that these positive emotions lasted after the sessions were completed and also increased over the course of the study. Additionally, analysis of the results indicated that these increased positive emotions also led to significant increases in several of the resources assessed, such as self-acceptance, purpose in life, and positive relations with others. In turn, analysis also demonstrated that these increases in positive resources led to increased life satisfaction. This study indicates that LKM can act as a catalyst for positive emotions, setting the broaden-and-build theory into motion and helping people enhance their well-being over time.

In another study using LKM, Fredrickson and colleagues sought to demonstrate the potential of positive emotions to have an impact on physical health in addition to psychological well-being by introducing the physiological measure of vagal tone (Kok et al. 2013). By measuring the variability of heart rate in conjunction with patterns of breathing, one can assess how well the vagus nerve is functioning (Porges 2007). The vagus nerve is the extension of the parasympathetic nervous system and returns the body, including a person's heart rate, to homeostasis. Low vagal tone has been linked to poor physical health, whereas high vagal tone has been associated with increased positive emotions (Bibevski and Dunlap 2011; Kok and Fredrickson 2010; Thayer and Sternberg 2006). In this particular study, Kok et al. (2013) wanted to see if it was possible to capture the upward spiral of positive emotions and good physical health using LKM. A sample of university employees were randomly assigned to either a 6-week LKM workshop or a control condition. Baseline vagal tone was measured prior to the intervention and again at the conclusion of the study. Participants also reported daily on their positive emotions, time spent meditating, and social interactions. After analysis, the results indicated that individuals in the LKM condition had increases in positive emotions and perceived social connectedness and higher vagal tone compared with the control group. These results provide additional support for the broaden-and-build theory and again demonstrate that LKM can increase experiences of positive emotions, which in turn increase psychological and physical well-being.

Further physiological evidence for the link between mindfulness and positive emotion has been gathered in a study examining brain function following a meditation program (Davidson et al. 2003). In this study, Mindfulness-Based Stress Reduction (MBSR) was used in the experimental condition as opposed to LKM. The researchers measured participants' brain activity using an electroencephalogram (EEG) and found that those who had completed the MBSR program had increased activation in the left-sided anterior cortex, which is consistent with patterns of activation in those exhibiting positive emotion (Davidson 1992; Davidson et al. 1990). This finding further supports meditation's ability to increase positive emotion; however, it goes even further by suggesting it does this by altering brain activity.

Other studies have also shown the connection between mindfulness and positive emotions. A year-long longitudinal study of physicians found that those who had attended an 8-week MBSR program had significant increases in mindfulness and positive emotional states, as well as significant decreases in

heart rate both directly after the intervention and also after a 10-month maintenance period (Amutio et al. 2015). Another study, this one using an 8-week
Mindfulness-Based Cognitive Therapy (MBCT) program with a nonclinical
sample, found that this program produced significant increases in positive affect, which were mediated by decreases in disengagement coping styles, such
as avoidance or denial (Cousin and Crane 2015). These findings provide additional evidence that mindfulness can facilitate the cultivation of positive emotions in individuals.

Although positive emotions might seem at first to be basic and obvious
components of well-being, their far-reaching and cumulative impact, as illus-
trated by the broaden-and-build theory and studies incorporating psychological
and physiological data, is actually much more nuanced and sophisticated.
These studies show that mindfulness, in various forms of meditation and training programs, can serve as a starting point for accessing and increasing positive
emotions, ultimately leading to greater gains in future well-being.

Engagement

Of the five elements of PERMA, perhaps none is more identified with a single
researcher, psychologist Mihály Csíkszentmihályi, than engagement (the E in
PERMA). Csíkszentmihályi lived through World War II in Hungary and became fascinated with why some of his family members remained more psycho-
logically intact while others sank into despair. He noticed that the people who
developed greater fortitude and tolerated life's challenges more successfully
had some activity in which their attention was completely absorbed, whether it
was chess, rock climbing, or the creation of art. They were so absorbed by the
activity that they seemed to lose track of time and did not report experiencing
any type of emotion but afterward were left invigorated by the experience.
Csíkszentmihályi named this type of experience *flow* (also known as *engagement* or *the zone*) and dedicated his life to studying its impact on athletes, great
thinkers, artists, and people in every domain of life.

Following more than 40 years of research, Csíkszentmihályi and colleagues
have developed several criteria for the achievement of flow (Nakamura and
Csikszentmihalyi 2009):

- Achievable challenge, meaning there must be a balance between the skills
  of the person and the challenge of the task, ideally with the challenge being
  slightly above the skill level of the participant
- Clear goals
- Immediate feedback (either internal or external)
- Focused attention

- A sense of autonomy or self-control
- A distorted sense of time (usually time passes quickly)

Csíkszentmihályi has studied the ability to achieve flow in a variety of occupations and pursuits and has found it to be consistently linked to well-being, self-esteem, role satisfaction, work productivity, and satisfaction with life (Emerson 1998). What is key to understanding flow is that it is not just "fun" and that not all activities involving focused attention can be categorized as flow. Watching TV, browsing the Internet, or playing video games can keep people mesmerized for hours but have been labeled as *junk flow*. A person does not watch 5 hours of a favorite sitcom, stand up and state, "Wow, that felt great!" The sense of competence, fulfillment, and productivity that one experiences with flow sets it apart from junk flow or simply having a good time. Another differentiation is that flow requires some degree of challenge, which is often not found in junk flow activities. In activities of junk flow, there is a quality of being passive; in contrast, true flow is a very active process, as is the practice of meditation and mindfulness.

On April 12, 2013, during grand rounds at the NYU Child Study Center, Csíkszentmihályi was asked if there is a relationship between flow—that moment of heightened attention and presence—and mindfulness meditation (Csíkszentmihályi (2013). His response was that meditation was like "bottled flow" and posited that it was the only experience of flow that he could imagine devoid of any activity outside of the person and his or her breath (Csíkszentmihályi 2013). In his response, Csíkszentmihályi highlighted the similarities between flow and mindfulness, a focusing of attention and presence in the moment. Indeed, research has suggested that developing mindfulness in one's life may allow people to experience greater amounts of flow as well.

Given the potential overlap of meditation, mindfulness, and the experience of flow, a number of clinicians and researchers have become interested in their relationship. There are many limitations in the research of mindfulness and flow because both are highly subjective experiences. For instance, research into flow has often involved the experience sampling method, in which a subject wears a pager that, when activated, signals the subject to write down his or her activity and the degree to which he or she is experiencing flow. Regardless of methodological research limitations, mindfulness and flow share many similarities. For example, in an attempt to operationalize mindfulness for the sake of research, Bishop et al. (2004) developed a definition of mindfulness as a psychological process that includes self-regulation of attention as well as a curiosity and acceptance of one's orientation to experience. This definition of mindfulness shares similarities with Csíkszentmihályi's characterization of flow, in that when people experience flow their attention is entirely absorbed by the process itself. Conversely, individuals with greater attention appear to experience more flow. In a study of the relationship between flow and attention in 240 undergraduates, Cermakova et al. (2010) found that those with greater capacity for attention experienced significantly more flow ($r=0.55$; $P<0.01$). The self-regulation of attention cultivated by mindfulness could potentially create increased opportunity for flow.

A few researchers are beginning to examine the relationship of how flow and mindfulness influence each other. In a study including 182 undergraduate athletes, Kee and Wang (2008) assessed both flow disposition and trait mindfulness. Students who were found to be high in mindfulness were also found to experience significantly more flow (Kee and Wang 2008). Additionally, the students high in mindfulness had more attentional and emotional self-regulation and were more inclined to use positive self-talk to bolster their efforts (Kee and Wang 2008). Being present and in the moment allows for a less judgmental relationship toward negative affect and potentially allows for greater resources, such as positive self-talk, to react appropriately to challenges.

In a similar but smaller intervention, 10 adult music students attended a series of yoga sessions to increase feelings of mindfulness and flow (Butzer et al. 2016). A control group of 15 students did not participate in the yoga program. The yoga group experienced an increase in both mindfulness and flow and a significant decrease in music performance anxiety. Playing music is regarded as being high in the experience of flow. The idea that developing flow in one area of a person's life (in this case yoga) may allow them to experience more flow in another (their music) could be an exciting avenue of future research and intervention.

Additional support for the connection between flow and mindfulness appears in a study by Moore (2013) on the relationship between mindfulness, cognitive flexibility, and increasing experiences of flow. Moore describes cognitive flexibility as an openness to new thoughts. In the study, he finds a correlation with greater flexibility and increased experience of flow. Just as Bishop et al. (2004) describe a central component of mindfulness as being open to experiences, Moore points out the value of cognitive flexibility to maintain states of flow. Flow requires feedback and adaptation as challenges increase. If one is resistant to these things, the experience of flow will be inhibited. Therefore, one way mindfulness may indirectly increase experiences of flow is by increasing cognitive flexibility.

The relationship between flow and mindfulness may be a neurological phenomenon as well. In a study of task performance, using EEG, Kramer (2007) found that both theta activity and greater alpha activity in the left temporal lobe were predictive of a flow state. Increased alpha and theta activity has also been seen in meditation as well (Cahn and Polich 2006).

Engagement is one of the essential components that Seligman (2011) prescribes for people to flourish in life. Helping a patient develop more flow may be successfully achieved by encouraging greater mindfulness. Yoga, meditation, or other activities that increase mindfulness and cognitive flexibility may be a prerequisite to fully experiencing flow. As Csíkszentmihályi (2013) has suggested, practitioners of meditation have the opportunity to carry a bottle of flow with them wherever they find themselves. While stuck in traffic, suffering through a boring lecture, or waiting for an elevator, practitioners can engage with their breath, improve their well-being, and take a sip of flow.

Positive Relationships

When asked to summarize positive psychology, Christopher Peterson, a founding figure in the field, succinctly stated, "Other people matter" (Peterson 2006). These three words are often invoked within the positive psychology community and underscore the importance of positive relationships, the R in PERMA. Positive psychology acknowledges that fostering relationships fulfills an innate human need. It also goes a step further to illustrate the potential of such relationships to contribute to increased well-being. Although the research on mindfulness and interpersonal relationships is in the early stages, mindfulness encourages openness and emotion regulation that can both fortify relationships and allow them to thrive.

Many of the studies examining the link between mindfulness and interpersonal relationships focus specifically on the relationships between spouses. One such study used survey data to look at the connection between mindfulness and marital satisfaction (Burpee and Langer 2005). The results showed a significant positive correlation between the two, meaning that participants who reported more frequent experiences of mindfulness were more likely to evaluate their relationship as satisfying. Possible reasons for this correlation could be that engaging in mindfulness allows for people to be more flexible in their approach to the relationship and their perception of their partner. The researchers suggest that the heightened awareness of the present moment cultivated by mindfulness could prevent recurring arguments by opening space for new interpretations of the circumstances instead of mindlessly repeating former patterns of conflicts. Additionally, because mindfulness is a constant practice, it might also stave off stagnation in the relationship by stemming the conversion of beloved rituals into monotonous habits.

The results of the study by Burpee and Langer (2005) also indicate that high marital satisfaction could be correlated with increased mindfulness because partners are less threatened by change, either in the relationship or in their partner. Therefore, the open-mindedness created by mindfulness has the potential to increase feelings of safety within the relationship, which could increase marital satisfaction. It is important to note that this study operationalized mindfulness using a conceptualization that focuses on looking for novel interpretations of the present moment instead of falling into the mindless routine of applying past patterns to current situations. The fact that this differs slightly from other definitions of mindfulness could impact the ability to generalize the results of Burpee and Langer's study to other applications of mindfulness. Also, because this is a correlational study, there is no way to know whether mindfulness causes high marital satisfaction or whether high marital satisfaction causes higher levels of mindfulness. Despite these shortcomings, the study does provide preliminary evidence that mindfulness and positive relationships are positively connected.

A separate study conducted using survey data found that mindfulness increases marital satisfaction by increasing spousal attachment (Jones et al. 2011). Increasing an individual's ability to focus his or her attention and awareness in nonjudgmental ways when interacting with his or her partner potentially increases the safety and security the partner feels within the relationship, thereby boosting the level of satisfaction. Although this study has several limitations, its results add additional support for the idea that mindfulness and positive relationships impact each other.

The study of a mindfulness-based relationship enhancement program, which incorporated interventions using elements of MBSR, LKM, yoga, and other activities integrating components of mindfulness, gave further evidence to support the use of mindfulness to enhance relationships (Carson et al. 2004). The couples participating in the study were screened to ensure that they entered the program without existing relationship troubles, and then they were randomly assigned to the experimental condition or to a waitlist control group. The program included 2½-hour weekly sessions for 8 weeks and a separate 6-hour retreat. On completion of the program, couples in the experimental condition had significantly improved their relationship satisfaction and also their relatedness to and acceptance of their partner.

Research on how mindfulness can impact relationships outside of the context of marriage also demonstrates a positive connection. In a study on helping behavior, researchers found that those participants who reported higher levels of present-focused attention and nonjudgmental acceptance reported greater helping behavior (Cameron and Fredrickson 2015). Engaging in such prosocial behavior could promote the initiation of new relationships and also foster existing relationships, thereby contributing to a person's overall well-being.

Although more research is needed to investigate the connections between mindfulness and a wider variety of relationships, the existing research indicates the potential of mindfulness to impact well-being through nurturing elements of positive relationships. Key aspects of mindfulness, such as increasing awareness of the present moment and remaining nonjudgmental and open-minded, allow people to be more attuned to those around them, potentially developing greater feelings of safety and satisfaction in their existing relationships and opening the door for creating new bonds as well. It seems that by engaging in mindfulness, people have more opportunities to discover just how much "other people matter."

Meaning

We characterize a meaningful life (represented by the M in PERMA) as comprising a person's comprehension of the world around him or her and the person's investment in a self-concordant purpose (Steger 2012). The importance of living "the good [or meaningful] life" can be traced back to Aristotle, who called this allegiance to one's inner virtues *eudaimonia* (Peterson 2006). In contrast to *hedonism*, or the singular pursuit of pleasure, eudaimonia describes cultivating one's best self and using it to serve a greater good. In modern research, meaning is "the web of connections, understandings and interpretations that help us comprehend our experience and formulate plans directing our energies to the achievement of our desired future" (Steger 2012, p. 2). Meaning provides a person with the feeling that his or her life is important and makes sense in the larger picture of what it means to be human.

In some theories, meaning or purpose in life is a definitional characteristic of well-being—that is, a person cannot be considered to have achieved well-being if he or she does not feel that his or her life has meaning or purpose. People who report greater meaning in their lives also report greater well-being, lesser psychopathology, and more beneficial experiencing of spirituality (Steger 2012).

Meaning can be cultivated in a variety of ways, one of which is through mindfulness. Although mindfulness practitioners have reported enhanced meaning in their lives for centuries, little research has sought to qualify these claims. An exception is a study by McGregor and Little (1998), who found that mindfulness practice leads to greater levels of perceived meaning in life. Ryan et al. (2008) theorized that people who have greater levels of mindfulness are less materialistic, embrace more intrinsic (relative to extrinsic) values, and experience less discrepancy between what they have and what they want and are therefore less dependent on external conditions for well-being.

The recently described *mindfulness-to-meaning theory* seeks to put a name to a phenomenon that practitioners have known all along, as well as to describe the mechanism that leads mindfulness to elicit a greater sense of meaning. Mindfulness facilitates greater meaning by allowing one to decenter from stress appraisals into a metacognitive state of awareness, resulting in broadened attention to novel information that accommodates a reappraisal of life circumstances. This reappraisal is then enriched when one savors positive features of the socioenvironmental context, subsequently motivating values-driven behavior and ultimately engendering eudaimonic meaning in life (Garland et al. 2015).

According to this model, the path to cultivating a sense of meaningfulness begins with a metacognitive monitoring of our experience without appraisal (i.e., nonjudgmentally). This nonjudgmental awareness is the very definition of mindfulness espoused by Jon Kabat-Zinn, which allows us to see and inhabit the space between stimulus and response (Kabat-Zinn 1990). In this model, that space is between a stressful event and how we appraise it. In creating this space, our attention broadens and makes room for a positive reappraisal of the event, ultimately facilitating greater positive emotion, savoring, and a sense of meaningfulness.

Accomplishment/Achievement

It may sound counterintuitive that mindfulness could have anything to do with accomplishment/achievement, which is the A in PERMA, but the locus of self-control that is developed through meditation and attention comes with an intrinsic sense of accomplishment. Seligman (2011) identified the need for achievement both extrinsically (e.g., money, fame, power) and intrinsically (e.g., a person's capacity as a parent, as a child, or in this case as a practitioner of meditation). Achievement has as much to do with external praise and concrete accomplishments as it does with feelings of competence, which has been identified in self-determination theory as an essential need. Both meditation and mindfulness can be thought of as skills, and their development, although very intrinsic, brings greater senses of self-control and mastery (Bishop et al. 2004).

In meditation, the expectation of reward and achievement is diminished in favor of developing the practice for its own intrinsic merits. Being overly preoccupied with the "payoff" inherently obstructs the development of attention (and mindfulness). The beginning practitioner is encouraged to relinquish attention on a specific achievement in favor of focusing intention on his or her breath or movement of the belly. If the student of meditation is truly focusing attention on his or her abdomen or breath, the development of concentration and emotion regulation will ultimately bring great benefit to the practitioner (and may lead to further achievements).

Although students of meditation are encouraged to relinquish expectations, there is great value placed on the practitioner's intentions. It is important to highlight the distinction between goals and intentions. A *goal* is an orientation toward a future desired outcome. Goals can be helpful to move one forward, but they can sometimes lead one to become preoccupied with the outcome, which is counterproductive when cultivating mindfulness. Setting an *intention*, however, is an orientation toward the *process* as opposed to the outcome. In meditation, instead of setting the *goal* to rid oneself of anxiety, one may instead set the *intention* to be nonjudgmental toward one's experience. This intention often leads to the goal of ridding oneself of anxiety. In contrast, when one sets the goal of ridding oneself of anxiety without developing any awareness of what is underlying it, relief, if any, is often short lived. In her research, Deane Shapiro (1992) observed that practitioners indeed set goals regarding self-regulation and stress management, which are reflected in these intentions.

Whether they have intentions or goals, practitioners of meditation and those who develop mindfulness do so for a reason. They develop greater attention, self-regulation, and positive emotions and may even experience greater amounts of flow in their life. As practitioners see the change that comes with developing mindfulness, they will develop the same locus of self-control that people who diet or exercise experience when they see their progress. Achievement may not be the goal of meditation, but it is certainly a benefit.

Conclusion

If Martin Seligman is one of the fathers of positive psychology, then Victor Frankl may be thought of as one of its grandfathers. Frankl was a psychiatrist steeped in the study and treatment of illness but was equally possessed by an interest in what makes humanity flourish. His area of interest was primarily the M of PERMA. He created a type of therapy focused entirely on helping people develop meaning in their life. He pushed his patients to find that space between stimulus and response, where a path toward growth can be found. Mindfulness allows patients to inhabit this space.

When Frankl gave a talk in May 1972 to the Toronto Youth Corps, he quoted the philosopher Goethe: "If we take man as he is, we make him worse, but if we take man as he should be, we make him capable of becoming what he can be" (Frankl 1972). Positive psychology gives the clinician a language to help patients comprehend what they can be and allows them to become capable of much more than what they are. Mindfulness and the practice of meditation may be a powerful way of inhabiting the elements of PERMA and enabling ourselves and our patients to aspire to something beyond the elimination of sickness. Mindfulness and meditation may enable us to develop positive emotions, engagement, positive relationships, meaning, and a sense of achievement.

Key Points for Further Study and Reflection

- Positive psychology is a growing field dedicated to the research and clinical application of well-being for our patients and society. One definition of well-being developed by Seligman (2011) involves individuals having sufficient PERMA—**P**ositive emotions, **E**ngagement, (positive) **R**elationships, **M**eaning, and **A**ccomplishment.

- Mindfulness and meditation are tools that can be used by both clinicians and patients to help them benefit from all aspects of PERMA. These practices have the potential to help people overcome challenges and also to develop greater well-being.

References

Amutio A, Martínez-Taboada C, Hermosilla D, Delgado LC: Enhancing relaxation states and positive emotions in physicians through a mindfulness training program: a one-year study. Psychol Health Med 20(6):720–731, 2015 25485658

Bibevski S, Dunlap ME: Evidence for impaired vagus nerve activity in heart failure. Heart Fail Rev 16(2):129–135, 2011 20820912

Bishop SR, Lau M, Shapiro S, et al: Mindfulness: a proposed operational definition. Clin Psychol Sci Pract 11(3):230–241, 2004

Burpee LC, Langer EJ: Mindfulness and marital satisfaction. J Adult Dev 12(1):43–51, 2005

Butzer B, Ahmed K, Khalsa SBS: Yoga enhances positive psychological states in young adult musicians. Appl Psychophysiol Biofeedback 41(2):191–202, 2016

Cahn BR, Polich J: Meditation states and traits: EEG, ERP, and neuroimaging studies. Psychol Bull 132(2):180–211, 2006 16536641

Cameron CD, Fredrickson BL: Mindfulness facets predict helping behavior and distinct helping-related emotions. Mindfulness (NY) 6:1211–1218, 2015

Carson JW, Carson KM, Gil KM, Baucom DH: Mindfulness based relationship enhancement. Behav Ther 35:471–494, 2004

Cermakova L, Moneta GB, Spada MM: Dispositional flow as a mediator of the relationships between attentional control and approaches to studying during academic examination preparation. Educ Psychol (Lond) 30(5):495–511, 2010

Cousin G, Crane C: Changes in disengagement coping mediate changes in affect following mindfulness-based cognitive therapy in a non-clinical sample. Br J Psychol Sept 19, 2015 DOI: 10.1111/bjop.12153 26385256, [Epub ahead of print]

Csíkszentmihályi M: Studying optimal experience: flow theory and research. Lecture given to the NYU Child Study Center, New York, April 12, 2013.

Davidson RJ: Emotion and affective style: hemisphere substrates. Psychol Sci 3:39–43, 1992

Davidson RJ, Ekman P, Saron CD, et al: Approach-withdrawal and cerebral asymmetry: emotional expression and brain physiology, I. J Pers Soc Psychol 58(2):330–341, 1990 2319445

Davidson RJ, Kabat-Zinn J, Schumacher J, et al: Alterations in brain and immune function produced by mindfulness meditation. Psychosom Med 65(4):564–570, 2003 12883106

Emerson H: Flow and occupation: a review of the literature. Can J Occup Ther 65(1):37–44, 1998

Frankl V: Why believe in others. Lecture given to the Toronto Youth Corps, Toronto, ON, Canada, May 1972. Available at: https://www.ted.com/talks/viktor_frankl_youth_in_search_of_meaning. Accessed March 15, 2016.

Frankl VE: Man's Search for Meaning (1946). New York, Simon & Schuster, 1985

Fredrickson BL: The role of positive emotions in positive psychology: the broaden-and-build theory of positive emotions. Am Psychol 56(3):218–226, 2001 11315248

Fredrickson BL: Positivity. New York, Three Rivers Press, 2009

Fredrickson BL, Mancuso RA, Branigan C, Tugade MM: The undoing effects of positive emotions. Motiv Emot 24(4):237–258, 2000 21731120

Fredrickson BL, Cohn MA, Coffey KA, et al: Open hearts build lives: positive emotions, induced through loving-kindness meditation, build consequential personal resources. J Pers Soc Psychol 95(5):1045–1062, 2008 18954193

Garland EL, Farb NA, Goldin P, Fredrickson BL: Mindfulness broadens awareness and builds eudaimonic meaning: a process model of mindful positive emotion regulation. Psychol Inq 26(4):293–314, 2015 27087765

Jones KC, Welton SR, Oliver TC, Thoburn JW: Mindfulness, spousal attachment, and marital satisfaction: a mediated model. Fam J (Alex Va) 19(4):357–361, 2011

Kabat-Zinn J: Full Catastrophe Living: Using the Wisdom of Your Body and Mind to Face Stress, Pain, and Illness. New York, Delacorte, 1990

Kee Y, Wang CJ: Relationships between mindfulness, flow dispositions and mental skills adoption: a cluster analytic approach. Psychol Sport Exerc 9(4):393–411, 2008

Kelly A: Gross national happiness in Bhutan: the big idea from a tiny state that could change the world. The Guardian 1(12), 2012

Kok BE, Fredrickson BL: Upward spirals of the heart: autonomic flexibility, as indexed by vagal tone, reciprocally and prospectively predicts positive emotions and social connectedness. Biol Psychol 85(3):432–436, 2010 20851735

Kok BE, Coffey KA, Cohn MA, et al: How positive emotions build physical health: perceived positive social connections account for the upward spiral between positive emotions and vagal tone. Psychol Sci 24(7):1123–1132, 2013 23649562

Kramer D: Predictions of performance by EEG and skin conductance. Indiana Undergraduate Journal of Cognitive Science 2:3–13, 2007

McGregor I, Little BR: Personal projects, happiness, and meaning: on doing well and being yourself. J Pers Soc Psychol 74(2):494–512, 1998 9491589

Mindful Schools: Online mindfulness training for educators. Available at: http://www.mindfulschools.org/. Accessed March 5, 2016.

Moore BA: Propensity for experiencing flow: the roles of cognitive flexibility and mindfulness. Humanist Psychol 41:319–322, 2013

Nakamura J, Csikszentmihalyi M: Flow theory and research, in The Oxford Handbook of Positive Psychology. Edited by Lopez SJ, Snyder CR. New York, Oxford University Press, 2009, pp 195–206

Pawelski JO, Moores DJ (eds): The Eudaimonic Turn: Well-Being in Literary Studies. Madison, NJ, Fairleigh Dickinson University Press, 2013

Peterson C: A Primer in Positive Psychology. New York, Oxford University Press, 2006, p 249

Pinsker J: Corporations' newest productivity hack: meditation. The Atlantic 10, 2015. Available at: http://www.theatlantic.com/business/archive/2015/03/corporations-newest-productivity-hack-meditation/387286/. Accessed February 10, 2016.

Porges SW: The polyvagal perspective. Biol Psychol 74(2):116–143, 2007 17049418

Ryan RM, Huta V, Deci EL: Living well: a self-determination theory perspective on eudaimonia. J Happiness Stud 9(1):139–170, 2008

Seligman ME: The president's address. Am Psychol 54(8):559–562, 1999

Seligman MEP: Flourish. New York, Atria Books, 2011

Shapiro DH: A preliminary study of long-term meditators: goals, effects, religious orientation, cognitions. J Transpers Psychol 24(1):23–39, 1992

Steger MF: Experiencing meaning in life: optimal functioning at the nexus of well-being, psychopathology, and spirituality, in The Human Quest for Meaning: Theories, Research, and Applications, 2nd Edition. Edited by Wong PTP. New York, Routledge/ Taylor & Francis, 2012, pp 165–184

Thayer JF, Sternberg E: Beyond heart rate variability: vagal regulation of allostatic systems. Ann NY Acad Sci 1088:361–372, 2006 17192580

Tony Hsieh, Chief Happiness Officer [video]. Time 2015. Available at: http://content.time.com/ time/specials/packages/article/0,28804,2091589_2092033_2099346,00.html?iid=sr-link1. Accessed February 8, 2016.

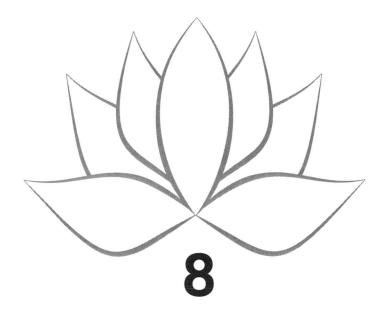

8

Promoting Mindfulness in Children and Adolescents

Mari Kurahashi, M.D., M.P.H.

My hope and wish is that one day, formal education will pay attention to what I call education of the heart. Just as we take for granted the need to acquire proficiency in the basic academic subjects, I am hopeful that a time will come when we can take it for granted that children will learn, as part of the curriculum, the indispensability of inner values: love, compassion, justice, and forgiveness.

The Dalai Lama,
Beyond Religion: Ethics for a Whole World

Mindfulness: The Evidence
With Children and Adolescents

In the recent mindfulness boom, enthusiasm has been shown for the use of mindfulness with children and adolescents. Part of the popularity of mindfulness for children and adolescents, as for adults, is based on research studies that support its multitude of purported benefits. These benefits include decreased anxiety, depression, attention-deficit/hyperactivity disorder, and substance abuse, in addition to improved general emotional well-being, academic performance, and emotion regulation. With these associated benefits, and many others, how could any parent or school be anything but on board with the mindfulness trend?

It is exciting that a practice that heralds from a more than 2,000-year-old Buddhist spiritual tradition is now secularized and widely practiced in the United States and abroad with scientific evidence to prove its effectiveness. However, as with the studies on mindfulness in adults, the excitement for the potential benefits of mindfulness practice in children may outweigh the actual evidence of its benefit because the quality of the studies is limited and the study results tend to show a low to moderate effect. Because of the relatively small number of studies done in children, as well as various limitations when doing research with children, the studies on mindfulness conducted with children and adolescents should be interpreted cautiously (Greenberg 2011). To improve their quality, mindfulness studies in general, as well as studies with children and adolescents, need to be randomized controlled trials (the gold standard of evidence-based medicine), have sufficient power, use validated and unbiased measures, have longer-term follow-up to measure the sustained impact of mindfulness, and include active control groups.

Studies also need to provide a clear description of the intervention being used because the many types of mindfulness practices, such as yoga, Mindfulness-Based Stress Reduction, Mindfulness-Based Cognitive Therapy, and Transcendental Meditation, are often lumped together under the broad umbrella of "mindfulness." These traditions use different techniques and have varying goals, however, so categorizing them together under the same label of "mindfulness" may complicate the data (Greenberg 2011). It is also important to acknowledge that these various practices often vary in duration, as well as the quality and duration of teacher training, which may have an impact on how mindfulness is learned and experienced by the research participants.

Despite the issues with mindfulness research in children and adolescents, there are certainly promising findings that are helpful in guiding mindfulness practices and research. Zoogman et al. (2014) conducted the first meta-analysis on mindfulness research with youth. They analyzed the literature from 2004 to 2011 and found that mindfulness interventions were helpful, with a small to moderate effect size, and were without iatrogenic harm. Interestingly, there was a significant increase in effect size when mindfulness practices were used with youth with psychological symptoms, when compared with their use in generally healthy participants who were recruited from schools.

Despite the limitations of validated and unbiased measures used in many of the studies, the participants overwhelmingly reported subjective enjoyment and improvements with their mindfulness practices, which is meaningful as well. Also, when parents participated in mindfulness practices as part of the mindfulness practice protocol for their children, the parents reported a subjective improvement in their own stress and anxiety, as well as in their children's symptoms. Improving the quality of the studies would help to ensure that the positive experiences and perceptions reported by the children and parents are due to mindfulness itself and to better understand how mindfulness works in affecting these symptoms and for which participants.

Potential Theories for Mindfulness and Its Impact on Children and Adolescents

There are many exciting potential benefits of introducing children and adolescents to mindfulness. One interesting theory involves the potential impact of the meditation "dose response." When an increase in an activity or medication dose has more effect than a lower level, this is called a *dose response* and can indicate cause and effect. Research shows that for monks and nuns with long-standing meditation practices, there is an association between longer and more advanced meditation practices and psychological well-being (Verma and Araya 2010). The underlying biological reason for this dose response is likely to be neuroplasticity, which is how the brain changes with experience. Scientists once believed that brain nerve cell connections were fixed early in life, but with brain imaging advances over the past two decades, scientists now widely accept the exciting idea of neuroplasticity, meaning that the brain continues to develop throughout one's life. Mindfulness may be a way to train the mind and impact neuroplasticity in the brain, similar to the way physical exercise improves physical health. Neuroscientist Richard Davidson conducted studies that showed that monks with long-standing meditation practices demonstrated differences in brain circuitry when compared with novice meditators (Lutz et al. 2004). He was particularly interested in gamma brain waves, which are involved in higher mental activities, such as perception and consciousness, and are critical in neuronal communication. Davidson found that monks with the longest meditation practices showed the highest levels of gamma wave activity. They also had higher amplitudes of gamma wave activity, which indicates a higher degree of synchronization of neuronal firing. This synchronized neuronal firing allows for improved communication between disparate brain nerve cells so the brain can function more efficiently. On the basis of this research and the notion of dose response, if children are exposed to meditation from a young age, there is the potential for them to experience a greater dose effect on their brain circuitry over time. At the same time, it is important to keep in mind that there is no clear evidence of the direct benefits of increased gamma wave activity, and the potential benefits are based on inferences that need to be further studied.

In addition to finding a dose response in the brain circuitry with mindfulness meditation, Davidson also found dose response changes in the brain anatomy with mindfulness meditation (Davidson and Lutz 2008). The brain consists of two major layers: gray matter and white matter. Gray matter is the layer of gray tissue that covers the inner white core. Gray matter consists of the nerve cell bodies and branching dendrites and is therefore the command and control center of the brain, whereas white matter consists of mostly nerve fibers with their myelin sheaths. Gray matter declines with age, and that decline may be a potential marker for brain atrophy. Davidson and Lutz found that long-standing meditation is associated with a decrease in the decline of gray matter and therefore a possible decrease in brain atrophy. An interesting consideration is the potential impact of mindfulness meditation on the brain anatomies of children and adolescents over time, especially in terms of the rate of decline of gray matter. However, these findings need to be further supported by other research findings to substantiate the association between increased meditation and decrease in gray matter decline.

Mindfulness and Young Children

Young children can be models for mindfulness in certain ways. They are usually completely absorbed with the present, not worrying about the past or the future. When they are playing, they are just playing. When they are eating, they are simply eating. When something doesn't go their way, they have a meltdown and are fully engaged with their emotions without any suppression, and then the storm passes and they are off to play without rumination about the negative experience they just had. Many more mindfulness studies are done in adults than in children, and there tends to be an assumption that mindfulness works similarly in children and adolescents as in older populations. Although there are likely many similarities, there are also important differences in how mindfulness works in children and in adults as a result of different developmental stages.

Early childhood is characterized by dramatic developments in self-regulation skills due to the vast growth of neural networks in the prefrontal cortex, which is the front part of the brain that is involved in attention, memory, and executive function. Developmental social cognitive neuroscience research indicates that self-regulation develops from a dynamic interaction between top-down regulatory processes and bottom-up influences (Zelazo and Lyons 2012). Top-down aspects of self-regulation are often studied under the category of executive function, which is an umbrella term for the regulation of cognitive processes, such as cognitive flexibility, inhibitory control, and working memory. Bottom-up influences include automatically elicited emotional reactions, such as stress and anxiety. The bottom-up raw emotional experiences may influence a child's ability to recruit the neural networks involved in top-down self-regulation.

Mindfulness training may help the development of self-regulation, especially in early childhood when self-regulation is particularly malleable because of pronounced neural plasticity, by increasing top-down processes while decreasing bottom-up influences. The purpose is not to suppress the bottom-up emotional experiences but rather to experience them without being reactive. Therefore, the bottom-up experience itself is not decreased, but its influence on behavior may be weakened. Mindfulness training with the emphasis on being present with moment-to-moment experiences can be a top-down exercise on focus and sustained attention. At the same time, mindfulness training with the emphasis on being focused on the present in a nonjudgmental manner can also be a bottom-up exercise on being present with one's emotions and the impact of those emotions. Being present in this way can calm some emotions by decreasing rumination. Therefore, because mindfulness targets both top-down and bottom-up processes, mindfulness training can be a way to strengthen the neural connection between the self-regulatory top-down processes located in the prefrontal cortex and the bottom-up emotional processes that are located in the limbic system, which can then support emotion regulation. Mindfulness training is unique because most other interventions that attempt to increase self-regulation target only top-down processes and therefore are more limited. Being exposed to mindfulness practices from a young age may thus help enhance this neural connection, which could then support emotion regulation across the lifespan.

Mindfulness and Adolescents

The word *adolescence* is derived from the Latin verb *adolescere*, which means "to grow up." Adolescence is therefore the transition period from childhood to adulthood. Psychoanalyst and author Louise J. Kaplan (1995) wrote, "Adolescence represents an inner emotional upheaval, a struggle between the eternal human wish to cling to the past and the equally powerful wish to get on with the future" (p. 21). This period consists of many challenges, including puberty and cognitive shifts that include increased introspection and self-awareness. These changes are often both exciting and overwhelming, as shown by the steep increase in psychiatric disorders during this time.

Not only do negative emotional states, such as anxiety, peak in prevalence during adolescence but adolescents experience these negative states in more extreme manners than adults do. At this time, when adolescents tend to experience intensely negative emotions, they also have a greater inclination to participate in risk-taking behavior. The neural correlates to this pairing of intense negative emotions with high-risk behaviors are being explored and may be due to the adolescent brain's hyperactive and relatively mature subcortical limbic system paired with a relatively immature regulatory prefrontal cortex, as shown by functional neuroimaging studies (Somerville et al. 2010). The adolescent subcortical limbic systems that are involved with processing emotions and sensitivity to potential rewards are hyperactive, which may explain why adolescents are disproportionately driven to incentive seeking behavior by environmental cues, regardless of the potential consequences. The prefrontal cortex that typically regulates these subcortical regions in adults has a later onset of maturation and therefore may function at immature levels during adolescence and may have less regulatory control over subcortical regions in adolescents than in adults (Somerville et al. 2010). Thus, the relative immaturity of the prefrontal cortex results in a deficient ability to control negative emotions, resulting in increased emotional outputs and decreased ability to control risky behaviors. The imbalance of the immature adolescent's prefrontal cortex with the mature subcortical systems, especially when compared with the child's brain, in which both systems are immature, and the adult's brain, in which both are mature, may help explain why adolescence is marked by intense emotions and risky behaviors.

Another factor that plays a role in adolescence as a period of risky behaviors is the heightened sensitivity of adolescents to negative and positive reinforcement models. With negative reinforcement, behavior is influenced by the avoidance of negative affective states, which in adolescents can entail substance use and other risky impulsive behaviors. Negative reinforcement is also related to many adolescents having low distress tolerance in that they may have poor abilities to persist in goal-directed behavior despite affective distress, which can then result in an increase in risky behaviors to avoid and escape negative affective states. With positive reinforcement, behavior is influenced by seeking positive affective states, and adolescents' increased sensitivity to potential rewards may lead to an increase in substance use and other risky impulsive behaviors. Therefore, both the positive reinforcement process of increased sensitivity to potential rewards and the negative reinforcement process of avoiding negative affects underlie adolescent risk behaviors. Adolescence is thereby an important stage during which interventions that target associative learning can be powerful in decreasing the conditioning that often persists and strengthens throughout adulthood.

Mindfulness training offers a way to impact associative learning by decoupling associations rather than by creating new associations (Brewer et al. 2013). The success of mindfulness training may be due to its emphasis on the person's nonjudgmental observation of his or her cravings, rather than the person's avoiding, distracting from, or succumbing to them, any of which can result in an increased tolerance to craving itself. Various stimuli can cause cravings to arise, but when a person is able to observe them in an accepting manner, rather than react to them, the previously learned associative links between craving and impulsive behaviors may become decoupled (Brewer et al. 2013). Similarly, rather than reacting to negative affective states, such as anxiety, in automatic and habitual ways, such as indulging or avoiding the affect, mindfulness can increase a person's ability to observe these negative affective states. With observing, rather than automatically reacting, there can be an increase of interaction with the process of feeling, and therefore the response can be more flexible and appropriate to the given situation. Mindfulness training may help adolescents by increasing their tolerance of the strong urges to indulge in risky and pleasurable behaviors and thereby decoupling the previously positively reinforced link between these urges and subsequent behavior. Mindfulness training can also increase adolescents' curious and accepting attitudes and awareness toward their negative affective states and thereby decrease their need for partaking in risky and/or impulsive behavior to relieve their negative affective states. Thus, the previously negatively reinforced link between negative affect and risky behavior can also be decoupled.

Child Development and Mindfulness

Despite the impressive canon of Buddhist texts and teachings, these sources contain little to no information on how mindfulness and meditation are experienced by and taught to children and adolescents. One of the many potential benefits from the Western embrace and study of the long-standing Eastern tradition of mindfulness is the exploration of developmental considerations involved in the use of mindfulness with children and adolescents. It will be fascinating to continue to uncover how developmental factors impact mindfulness and how mindfulness impacts development in children and adolescents. As discussed earlier in the section "Potential Theories for Mindfulness and Its Impact on Children and Adolescents," one potential way to understand these developmental factors is through neuroscience. The following section on how to work with children and mindfulness has been informed by Western developmental and attachment theories. Ongoing study on how development may impact mindfulness can lead to continual improvements in establishing the most effective ways to teach and apply mindfulness with children and adolescents.

Working With Children and Mindfulness

A commonly used term within the mindfulness tradition is *child's mind*. This term describes what comes to mind when one reflects on a sweet memory from one's own childhood and considers how as a child one perceived the world and experiences. This child's mind is an important goal of mindfulness and is a reminder that when working with children, we are bringing out what is already inherently present in the child. We are encouraging the child's natural state of openness and receptivity. This child's mind comes naturally for a child and then, over time, becomes conditioned out because of an emphasis in education on analysis and categorization, so that there is a loss of the childlike tendency to be present without a filter of preconceived ideas. Therefore, when working with children, we need to remember that it may be easier for them to tap into experiencing the world with fresh, open, and curious eyes rather than with preconceived concepts. Children may serve as an inspiration for us as adults to find our way back to a child's mind.

Many mindfulness exercises for children embrace a fun activity-based focus to help break away from the tendency to analyze and conceptualize (Greenland 2010; Willard 2010). Activities such as playing instruments, dancing, blowing bubbles, playing interactive games, and making art can be used to introduce a mindfulness session. Hands-on demonstrations to illustrate mindfulness in a more experiential manner tend to be more effective for children and adolescents than are wordy cognitive explanations of mindfulness. Because of the shorter attention span of most children and adolescents, a general rule of thumb is to practice a mindfulness exercise for 1 minute per age of the child (e.g., 5 minutes for a 5-year-old). It can also be helpful to place mindfulness within the context of the child's goals and interests rather than to focus on the instructor's goals. For example, mindfulness practices by famous athletes and musicians may be more helpful in inspiring and motivating younger populations than speaking about the Buddha or famous nuns and monks. It is also important to emphasize that mindfulness is not about improving or changing problems within the child but rather is about adding onto the existing strengths that the child already possesses.

Consistency and routine are important for children in general, and this premise remains true with mindfulness practice (Greenland 2010; Willard 2010). Therefore, having a consistent time and place for mindfulness meditation can be helpful. Potential regular times may be after waking up, before going to sleep, before or after meals, at moments when the family is together, and at the start and end of therapy or mindfulness sessions. Whether one is teaching mindfulness to a group of children or to an individual child, working together to decorate a meditation space can be a way to connect and to establish a specific place for focusing on practicing mindfulness.

Although parents, teachers, and therapists may be tempted to remind children to use mindfulness skills when the children are displaying negative behaviors, the adults need to refrain from doing so because of the risk that the children will associate mindfulness with punishment (Greenland 2010; Willard 2010). Instead, when children practice mindfulness in general and not necessarily during difficult times, they are able to build up their mindfulness muscles and become better able to avoid or manage difficult situations. Rather than directing children while they are having difficulties, it is essential for caretakers to model mindfulness for the children during difficult situations without being reactive to their own difficult emotions. During these difficult episodes, caretakers often become upset and reactive or feel overwhelmed and closed off. Instead, they can acknowledge and experience the negative emotions in a curious, nonjudgmental manner and perhaps count their breaths individually or with the child.

The currently established Western mindfulness protocols for children and adolescents involve modifications that take into account developmental considerations (Greenland 2010; Willard 2010). In general, because of the more limited attention spans of children and adolescents, the sessions and length of meditation exercises are shorter in duration; however, the number of sessions is increased to compensate for the shorter durations. Parent involvement is common so that parents practice similar skills and can model, teach, and discuss the skills with their children. The hope is that these approaches can be adapted into the family culture for sustained benefits. Mindfulness-Based Stress Reduction has been modified for teens to focus on adolescent-specific stressors, such as social issues (Biegel 2009).

It is essential that providers establish their own practice of mindfulness before teaching mindfulness to children and adolescents. This is especially important in an era in which manualized treatments are often supported by research and are presented as being simple to follow. Mindfulness is largely experiential, and for providers to fully understand mindfulness, it is much more critical for them to develop their own practice than to learn about it cognitively. Only through having their own meditation practice can providers be able to fully connect with children's experiences and be able to help them in a more meaningful and insightful way. In addition, having their own practice will help providers conduct themselves in helpful ways, such as by not enforcing their own goals, intentions, and expectations and instead being open to the children's goals and perceptions. An individual regular practice will also allow a provider to speak, listen, and behave mindfully, all of which are critical behaviors for the provider to model for the children.

Mindfulness and Psychopathology

The first and only published meta-analysis on mindfulness interventions in youth was conducted by Zoogman et al. (2014). The general conclusion was that mindfulness interventions may be more helpful for youth with psychopathology symptoms, as indicated by a significantly larger effect size. This finding is important given the high prevalence of psychopathology in youth. Merikangas et al. (2009) reported that about 25% of youth in the United States experienced a mental health disorder in the previous year and estimated that about one-third will experience a mental health disorder within their lifetime. Notably, 70% of these adolescents with psychopathology do not receive care (Schwarz 2009) because of the limited number of treatments and even more limited access to existing treatments. Common reasons for the limited access to care include lack of adequate insurance coverage and the limited number of mental health providers who treat children and adolescents.

Even when youth have access to care, the most common evidence-based treatments for childhood psychopathology are psychotherapy and psychotropic medications. There are many concerns about treating children with psychotropic medications. Although medications can be helpful in treating many childhood psychopathologies, these treatments also have significant limitations and can have adverse effects as well. With psychotherapy, there is a range in effectiveness because of the wide variety of methods used and differences in the quality of the treatments. Even with the most evidence-based therapy, cognitive-behavioral therapy (CBT), there are limitations in its effectiveness and sustainability of its benefits. There are some parallels between mindfulness-based therapies and CBT, and some mindfulness-based therapies such as Mindfulness-Based Cognitive Therapy even incorporate some CBT elements.

What sets mindfulness-based therapies apart from CBT, however, is the focus in mindfulness-based therapies on being present with whatever is happening in an open, curious, and accepting manner. Conversely, in CBT, there is an intentional focus on analysis and change, usually on what is called the underlying cognitive distortion, in the hope that the individual can change his or her emotions and behaviors. With mindfulness, there is less effort in implementing change and more of an emphasis on tapping into a natural way of being. This practice then allows one to disconnect from the automatic and reactive loops of the thought processes and behaviors that are habitually engaged so that one can make calm and healthy decisions and experience life more fully.

Because of the limitations of conventional treatments, alternative psychiatric treatments, such as mindfulness, are needed. The benefits to mindfulness as a complementary treatment for childhood psychopathology are that it can be administered in a large-scale manner and can address the access limitations of conventional individual therapies. With their broad-scale application, especially in schools, mindfulness-based therapies can also be used as preventative and early intervention modalities of treatment. In addition, all the studies of mindfulness in youth have indicated its safety. There have been reports of adverse effects from intense meditation in adults, but there are no known reports of adverse effects from mindfulness-based therapies in youth, although this possibility should be continuously monitored.

Key Points for Further Study and Reflection

- There is substantial promising evidence for the benefits of mindfulness in children and adolescents, although better-quality studies are needed.
- It is important for providers to consider developmental factors when teaching mindfulness to children.
- Western psychology can contribute to traditional Buddhist psychology by elucidating how developmental factors impact the ways that mindfulness is taught to and experienced by children.
- Because of the prevalence of psychopathology in children and adolescents, as well as the limited access to care, mindfulness practice may be both an important treatment and a preventative measure.

References

Biegel GM: The Stress Reduction Workbook for Teens: Mindfulness Skills to Help You Deal With Stress. Oakland, CA, New Harbinger, 2009

Brewer JA, Elwafi HM, Davis JH: Craving to quit: psychological models and neurobiological mechanisms of mindfulness training as treatment for addictions. Psychol Addict Behav 27(2):366–379, 2013 22642859

Davidson RJ, Lutz A: Buddha's brain: neuroplasticity and meditation. IEEE Signal Process Mag 25(1):176–174, 2008 20871742

Greenberg M: Nurturing mindfulness in children and youth: current state of research. Child Dev Perspect 6(2):161–166, 2011

Greenland S: The Mindful Child: How to Help Your Kid Manage Stress and Become Happier, Kinder and More Compassionate. New York, Atria Books, 2010

Kaplan L: Adolescence: The Farewell to Childhood. New York, Touchstone Books, 1995

Lutz A, Greischar LL, Rawlings NB, et al: Long-term meditators self-induce high-amplitude gamma synchrony during mental practice. Proc Natl Acad Sci USA 101(46):16,369–16,373, 2004 15534199

Merikangas KR, Nakamura EF, Kessler RC: Epidemiology of mental disorders in children and adolescents. Dialogues Clin Neurosci 11(1):7–20, 2009 19432384

Schwarz SW: Adolescent mental health in the United States. New York, National Center for Children in Poverty, 2009. Available at www.nccp.org/publications/pub_878.html. Accessed July 15, 2016.

Somerville LH, Jones RM, Casey BJ: A time of change: behavioral and neural correlates of adolescent sensitivity to appetitive and aversive environmental cues. Brain Cogn 72(1):124–133, 2010 19695759

Verma G, Araya R: The effect of meditation on psychological distress among Buddhist monks and nuns. Int J Psychiatry Med 40(4):461–468, 2010 21391415

Willard C: Child's Mind: Mindfulness Practices to Help Our Children Be More Focused, Calm and Relaxed. Berkeley, CA, Parallax Press, 2010

Zelazo D, Lyons K: The potential benefits of mindfulness training in early childhood: a developmental social cognitive neuroscience perspective. Child Dev Perspect 6(2):154–160, 2012

Zoogman S, Goldberg S, Hoyt W, Miller L: Mindfulness interventions with youth: a meta-analysis. Mindfulness 6:290–302, 2014

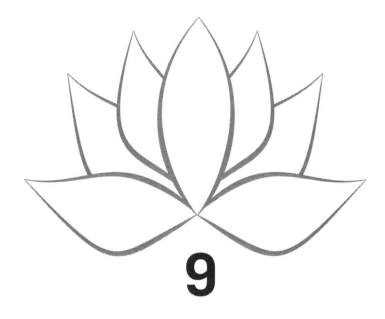

9

Mindfulness-Based Interventions for Substance Use Disorder Treatment

Allison K. Ungar, M.D.
Oscar G. Bukstein, M.D., M.P.H.

Radical acceptance rests on letting go of the illusion of control and a willingness to notice and accept things as they are right now, without judging.

Marsha M. Linehan

SUBSTANCE USE DISORDERS (SUDs) are prevalent and cause substantial morbidity and mortality. Along with other mental disorders, SUDs constitute the fifth leading cause of death and disability across the globe (Whiteford et al. 2013). SUDs are known to be clinically challenging to treat, and seasoned clinicians often find a need to integrate a number of different evidence-based therapeutic interventions to address their clients' needs. Mindfulness-based interventions (MBIs), defined as therapeutic techniques that employ a purposeful and nonjudgmental awareness of each moment, have demonstrated a growing evidence base (Chiesa and Serretti 2014). Clinical implementation of MBIs can be straightforward, and some MBIs have been manualized to make them easier to use. In this chapter, we aim to elaborate on the evidence base for various MBIs in treating SUDs and describe easily accessible means to take advantage of this treatment modality.

Mechanism of Action

From a biological and phenomenological perspective, addictions are disorders of learning and memory that have altered the salience of cues in the mesolimbic reward system. MBIs can be thought to hone skills in "top-down" control from the prefrontal cortex, allowing for improved inhibitory control over subcortical regions and historically rewarding behaviors (Rösner et al. 2015). Functional neuroimaging studies appear to support mindfulness being associated with an increased ability to dampen reactivity to craving-related cues (Westbrook et al. 2013). Westbrook and colleagues used functional magnetic resonance imaging to examine the neural activity of 47 smokers who were 12 hours abstinent from smoking. Participants were shown neutral images and images of smoking and were trained to view images either passively or mindfully. Mindful attention was associated with subjective reductions in craving and decreased neural activity in and connectivity to the craving-related brain structures, notably, the subgenual anterior cingulate cortex.

Being that MBIs are techniques that retrain the brain, it seems logical that people who practice these techniques will reap the neurocognitive benefits. In studying Mindfulness-Based Relapse Prevention (MBRP), a type of MBI, it has been found that individuals who increased home mindfulness practice had significantly lower alcohol and drug use, along with lower craving scores (Grow et al. 2015). This suggests that although mindfulness is effective, it requires ongoing enactment to support recovery. This provides credence to the clinical recommendation of practicing mindfulness on a daily basis rather than implementing techniques solely within high-risk situations.

In addition, in several mindfulness-directed tasks (e.g., mindful walking, mindful eating, awareness of breath, body scanning), the individual also develops the skill of being able to shift attention from a constant stream of unconsciousness back to the task at hand. This entrained ability to shift from a ruminating thought back to the sensations of the body can be utilized in the setting of cue-induced cravings.

Practicing mindfulness can also be thought to extinguish operantly and classically conditioned behaviors intrinsic to addiction. Mindfulness decouples learned behaviors from their associated memories by bringing nonjudgmental descriptive consciousness to previously subconscious cravings and behaviors (Brewer et al. 2013).

Benefits of Mindfulness in Treating Substance Use Disorders

Relapse

In treating SUDs, clinicians can use MBIs to assist their patients in dealing with noxious affective states that often trigger relapse. Conceptually, in bringing awareness to the present moment, the patient can make more mindful behavioral choices that are consistent with values and goals (e.g., choosing to remain abstinent from illicit drugs, alcohol, and nicotine). Traditional relapse prevention focuses on avoidance or minimization of triggers. Notably, because SUD triggers are ubiquitous, avoidance and mental diversion are both taxing and ineffective. Alternatively, MBIs do not strive to minimize triggers; rather, they bring nonjudgmental awareness to thoughts, feelings, and sensations in these situations. MBIs seek to disconnect the experience of a craving from the automatic response of substance use. Viktor Frankl has described the creation of this mindful state: "In between stimulus and response, there is a space. In that space lies our freedom and power to choose our response. In our response lies our growth and freedom" (Nelson 2005, p. 62).

Managing relapse remains an intrinsic aspect of treating the chronic nature of SUDs because 40%–60% of patients will experience a relapse in their treatment course (McLellan et al. 2000). Therefore, investigators have sought to demonstrate the sustained treatment effect of MBIs. Longitudinal studies of MBRP have demonstrated statistically and clinically significant effects for 12 months in reducing days of substance use and heavy drinking, as compared with both traditional relapse prevention and treatment as usual (TAU; Bowen et al. 2014). Longitudinal studies of acceptance and commitment therapy (ACT) for tobacco use disorder have also demonstrated clinical improvement at the 1-year mark as compared with nicotine replacement therapy (Gifford et al. 2004).

Relapses are nearly inevitable, which creates opportunities to apply a non-judgmental stance. With growing self-awareness, patients can begin to recognize when they have slipped back into old modes of thought and behavior.

Shame

SUDs are laden with the language of shame, regret, and fear. People suffering from SUDs are often humiliated by the limited remains of the life they once had, are mortified by behaviors inconsistent with their values that were done under the influence, and have a deep-seated pain about the effects of their substance use on their loved ones. This cognitive preoccupation and negative affect state lead to avoidance behaviors to minimize distress, such as treatment dropout and relapse. Patients may also try to suppress their shame, which can rebound with amplification.

> **Example of the cognitive rebound effect:** Don't think of a purple elephant!

> **The resultant experience:** You immediately imagine a purple elephant and have a hard time forgetting about that elephant. The harder you try to forget, the more the elephant appears in your stream of consciousness.

Luoma and colleagues (2012) explored shame as a modifiable factor through the use of ACT (for further discussion, see the subsection "Acceptance and Commitment Therapy" later in the chapter). They studied a population within a 28-day rehabilitation facility, comparing TAU with ACT. The ACT group demonstrated greater follow-up and less substance use, variables determined to be mediated by gradual reductions in shame. Mindfulness techniques loosen rigid self-constructs through use of descriptive rather than judgmental statements. This sort of language shift de-escalates the power of a thought (i.e., thoughts are not facts). The descriptive semantics can leave therapeutic space for objectivity and the development of self-compassion.

> **Example of a ruminating shameful thought:** "I cannot get sober. I always screw up. I am going to screw up again. I'm such a screw-up."

> **Employing a nonjudgmental mindful stance:** "I'm having the thought that I cannot get sober."

Cravings

In addition to addressing shame, MBIs are well suited to targeting cravings for drugs and alcohol. Cravings are often cited as the reason for relapse, although cravings are a difficult subjective experience for patients to describe and for clinicians to treat. Clinicians utilize relapse prevention skills such as avoiding people, places, and things that trigger substance use. Alternatively, MBIs seek to have patients tolerate uncomfortable affect states in these situations and engage in "urge surfing" on the natural crests and troughs of a craving (Marlatt and Gordon 1985). The goal of urge surfing is to "ride the wave" of thoughts, feelings, sensations, and external cues, without responding with a behavior. By not fighting with the craving, the client can avoid a "wipeout" (being overwhelmed by the feeling and subsequently engaging in substance use). In this mindful stance, patients can discover that cravings are transient physical sensations rather than "moral imperatives" that must be acted on (Brewer et al. 2013).

Investigators studying MBRP found this intervention to significantly decrease craving scores in comparison to a TAU control group (Witkiewitz et al. 2013). The decreased cravings were related to decreased substance use, mediated by increased acceptance, awareness, and a nonjudgmental attitude.

Example 1: Mindfully Sitting With a Craving

Clinician: Describe the present sensation of your craving without judgment.

Patient: There is the taste of the cocaine dripping down my throat, my heart is skipping a beat, my head is getting light, and the craving sensation is sitting in the pit of my stomach. I am having the thought "Just a little will make this discomfort go away."

Franz Kafka has described how the painful striving to escape suffering (e.g., cravings) leads to the pain itself. He states, "You can hold back from suffering of the world, you have permission to do so, and it is in accordance with your nature, but perhaps this very holding back is the one suffering you could have avoided" (Goldstein 2009).

Example 2: The Monster in the Room

Comical imagery can be used clinically to describe the change in one's relationship one's thoughts and feelings.

Situation 1: A child is fearful of the furry monster that lives under her bed. She checks to make sure that the monster is not there every time she enters her bedroom, which gives her momentary relief. She seeks reassurance repeatedly from her parents, who temporarily assuage her distress with warm milk.

Situation 2: The child recognizes that a furry monster lives in her room. She says, "Hello, Mr. Monster, would you like some tea?" The child proceeds with her make-believe tea party, acknowledging that she has another guest. Because the child is not upset by the presence of the unpleasant guest, the tea party is not disrupted.

Situation 1 applied to SUDs: An individual with alcohol use disorder is attending a work function. Anxiety streams through his body, his heart races, his hands sweat, and his fingers begin to tingle. The thought "I can't do this" streams repeatedly through his consciousness. The individual reaches for a flask in his pocket and takes a gulp of liquor, and the anxious thoughts and sensations dampen.

Situation 2 applied to SUDs: The individual with alcohol use disorder has the identical affective, physical, and cognitive experiences found in situation 1. He states, "I am having the thought that I cannot do this." He notices the physical sensations (heart racing, sweating, and tingling fingers) and names each experience without judgment. He then proceeds into the work function without attempts to suppress or change the experience.

Mindfulness-Based Interventions for Substance Use Disorders

Mindfulness has been formulated into a number of clinically effective interventions for treating SUDs, several of which will be reviewed herein. Multiple systematic reviews have been published on this topic (Chiesa and Serretti 2014; Zgierska et al. 2009). A Cochrane review is anticipated to further clarify the evidence strength of MBIs (Rösner et al. 2015).

Chiesa and Serretti (2014) provide a comprehensive review of the literature published until December 2011. In their examination of 24 MBI studies, the authors determined that MBIs have demonstrated efficacy across substance use disorders, including alcohol, stimulants (cocaine, methamphetamines), cannabis, opiates, and nicotine. Of note, MBIs are accessible in both online and in-person formats and are appropriate for special populations such as individuals with a low education level (Davis et al. 2015). Additionally, features of the MBIs can complement other SUD treatment modalities.

Acceptance and Commitment Therapy

ACT is a mindfulness-based behavioral therapy that utilizes an eclectic mix of metaphor, mindfulness skills, experiential exercises, and value-guided behavioral interventions (Hayes et al. 1999). It can be described as engagement in value-based activities with an awareness and willingness to experience the potentially distressing experience that may occur (e.g., thoughts, feelings, sensations, memories), which is termed *psychological flexibility*. ACT does not strive to challenge beliefs, stop pain, or analyze what went wrong. In SUDs, ACT can be thought to target experiential avoidance that occurs with ruminations of failures and fears of repeated mistakes.

ACT is based on a six-pronged model:

1. Being present—focusing on the here and now
2. Acceptance—being willing to experience difficult thoughts
3. Diffusion—observing thoughts without being ruled by them
4. Self as context—being unchanged by experiences
5. Values—discovering what is important to a person
6. Commitment—taking action to pursue the valued things in life

Example of an ACT Metaphor (modified from Hayes et al. 1999):

Monsters on a Bus

You are a bus driver, and you have many noisy monster riders coming along with you. These riders are thoughts, feelings, sensations, and memories. They shout profanities, throw spit balls at the back of your head, pull the emergency brake unnecessarily, open the window in the pouring rain, and simultaneously tell you that you are the worst driver they have ever had while threatening your physical safety. You could stop the bus and attend to all of the nuisances and clamor, but if you stop the bus, you would never make it to your destination on time and would not get paid. If you were to attempt to get control of your passengers, you would lose control over getting to your end goal.

Translation of Monsters on a Bus to the Treatment of SUDs

You are newly sober from alcohol, just home from a 3-month residential rehabilitation, and you are returning to work. You are a loving parent of three children who need food on the table. You know when you go to your job, people will ask where you have been, and there is going to be an expectation of joining the postwork happy hour. You say to yourself, "I am having the thought that I will be judged harshly." You notice a knot in your stomach and a feeling of nausea. You go to work because you value providing for your loved ones.

As mentioned previously, ACT has evidence for reducing measures of shame (Luoma et al. 2012) and for treating multiple SUDs (Chiesa and Serretti

2014). In a meta-analysis of ACT for treating SUDs, Lee et al. (2015) demonstrated a small to medium effect size supporting ACT. Of particular clinical relevance is ACT's efficacy in treating cannabis and stimulant use disorders, which do not currently have any available pharmacological treatments approved by the U.S. Food and Drug Administration. ACT has also been used successfully with unique populations such as incarcerated women (Lanza et al. 2014).

Dialectical Behavioral Therapy (DBT)

DBT is a 1-year manualized treatment program that is based on behavioral psychology, mindfulness practices, and a dialectical philosophy. DBT is delivered in individual and group settings along with a phone consultation setting. The "dialectic" is to live in the space and balance between two opposing forces: change and acceptance. Patients with SUDs have a strong desire to want to eradicate all distressing experiences, sometimes including life itself. This negative affect state must be tolerated in order to achieve a life worth living (consistent with the aforementioned value-driven behaviors of ACT). Within the DBT program, there are modules teaching mindfulness skills, distress tolerance, and radical acceptance. Consistent with other MBIs, DBT seeks to bring awareness to behaviors that may be dangerous, treatment interfering, or inconsistent with life goals (Dimeff and Linehan 2008).

In a randomized controlled trial, Linehan et al. (1999) compared DBT with TAU in polysubstance users with borderline personality disorder. The DBT group was less likely to drop out of treatment and had a higher proportion of drug and alcohol abstinence, with a treatment effect seen at 16-month follow-up. A second randomized controlled trial examined DBT versus comprehensive validation therapy with 12 steps in a population of opioid users on opioid replacement therapy. Although both groups demonstrated decreased drug use over the year-long study, only the DBT group maintained those gains in the last 4 months of the study (Linehan et al. 2002).

Mindfulness-Based Relapse Prevention

MBRP is a manualized aftercare intervention for SUD relapse prevention that integrates mindfulness-based stress reduction and mindfulness-based cognitive therapy. MBRP trains participants to recognize triggers, increase awareness of cravings, and mindfully accept uncomfortable physical and affective states (Bowen et al. 2011). MBRP has demonstrated efficacy in reducing cravings (Witkiewitz et al. 2013) and decreasing substance use as compared with TAU (Bowen et al. 2009).

A large (n=286) 1-year randomized controlled trial performed by Bowen and colleagues (2014) examined the efficacy of MBRP for aftercare as compared with TAU and cognitive-behavioral relapse prevention (CBRP), with primary outcomes of frequency of substance use in the last 90 days and heavy drinking days. The authors noted that CBRP was chosen as an empirically supported control condition. At the 6-month point CBRP and MBRP proved superior to TAU, although at 12 months MBRP and CBRP diverged in efficacy, with MBRP demonstrating longer-term superiority. The MBRP group had 31% fewer days of substance use than did the CBRP group and a higher probability of not having heavy drinking days.

12-Step Literature

Although 12-step-based interventions are not technically MBIs, in some ways their tenets are reflective of a mindful and acceptance-based stance. The serenity prayer said at every meeting uses language of acceptance. This prayer, written by Reinhold Niebuhr, is as follows: "God, grant me the serenity to accept the things I cannot change, the courage to change the things I can, and the wisdom to know the difference" (Shapiro 2014). In fact, the first of the 12 steps is that of radical acceptance and surrender in order to move successfully through the remaining steps (Alcoholics Anonymous World Services, Inc. 2001). In their review of MBIs, Chiesa and Serretti (2014) present data on several studies that use 12-step programs as the comparison group.

MBIs for Clinicians Treating Substance Use Disorders

Clinicians are also vulnerable to the downfalls of fixed cognitive and behavioral patterns. Although there are evidence-based pharmacological interventions for SUDs, only a limited percentage of patients receive the medications that are indicated for their diagnosis. There is a reluctance to try new pharmacotherapies—possibly a judgment of old being better than new or an underlying fear of the unknown.

Varra and colleagues (2008) examined the effectiveness of ACT for improving drug and alcohol counselors' provision of evidence-based agonist and antagonist pharmacotherapy for SUDs. They randomly asssigned 59 counselors to either a 1-day ACT workshop or a 1-day educational control workshop. Subsequently, both groups attended a 2-day seminar on empirically supported treatments for SUDs. Those in the ACT condition had higher rates of referrals to pharmacotherapy at a 3-month follow-up time point and fewer perceived barriers to trying new treatment interventions. The researchers posit that psychological flexibility on the clinicians' part may contribute to SUD treatment success.

Key Points for Further Study and Reflection

- Mindfulness-based interventions (MBIs) are helpful for treating many facets of substance use disorders, including shame from drug use, craving for continued use, and prevention of relapse.
- Several evidence-based MBIs are effective for treating substance use disorders, including acceptance and commitment therapy, dialectical behavioral therapy, and Mindfulness-Based Relapse Prevention.
- The psychological flexibility taught in MBIs may be helpful to clinicians in adopting evidence-based treatments.

References

Alcoholics Anonymous World Services, Inc.: Alcoholics Anonymous, Fourth Edition. New York, Alcoholics Anonymous World Services, 2001

Bowen S, Chawla N, Collins SE, et al: Mindfulness-based relapse prevention for substance use disorders: a pilot efficacy trial. Subst Abus 30(4):295–305, 2009 19904665

Bowen S, Chawla N, Marlatt GA: Mindfulness-Based Relapse Prevention for Addictive Behaviors: A Clinician's Guide. New York, Guilford, 2011

Bowen S, Witkiewitz K, Clifasefi SL, et al: Relative efficacy of mindfulness-based relapse prevention, standard relapse prevention, and treatment as usual for substance use disorders: a randomized clinical trial. JAMA Psychiatry 71(5):547–556, 2014 24647726

Brewer JA, Elwafi HM, Davis JH: Craving to quit: psychological models and neurobiological mechanisms of mindfulness training as treatment for addictions. Psychol Addict Behav 27(2):366–379, 2013 22642859

Chiesa A, Serretti A: Are mindfulness-based interventions effective for substance use disorders? A systematic review of the evidence. Subst Use Misuse 49(5):492–512, 2014 23461667

Davis JM, Manley AR, Goldberg SB, et al: Mindfulness training for smokers via web-based video instruction with phone support: a prospective observational study. BMC Complement Altern Med 15:95, 2015 25886752

Dimeff LA, Linehan MM: Dialectical behavior therapy for substance abusers. Addict Sci Clin Pract 4(2):39–47, 2008 18497717

Gifford EV, Kohlenberg BS, Hayes SC, et al: Acceptance-based treatment for smoking cessation. Behav Ther 35(4):689–705, 2004

Goldstein E: The one suffering you could avoid: Mondays mindful quote. Newburyport, MA, Psych Central, 2009. Available at: http://blogs.psychcentral.com/mindfulness/2009/11/the-one-suffering-you-could-avoid-mondays-mindful-quote/. Accessed July 4, 2016.

Grow JC, Collins SE, Harrop EN, Marlatt GA: Enactment of home practice following mindfulness-based relapse prevention and its association with substance-use outcomes. Addict Behav 40:16–20, 2015 25218066

Hayes SC, Strosahl KD, Wilson KG: Acceptance and Commitment Therapy: An Experiential Approach to Behavior Change. New York, Guilford, 1999

Lanza PV, García PF, Lamelas FR, González-Menéndez A: Acceptance and commitment therapy versus cognitive behavioral therapy in the treatment of substance use disorder with incarcerated women. J Clin Psychol 70(7):644–657, 2014 24449031

Lee EB, An W, Levin ME, Twohig MP: An initial meta-analysis of acceptance and commitment therapy for treating substance use disorders. Drug Alcohol Depend 155:1–7, 2015 26298552

Linehan MM, Schmidt H 3rd, Dimeff LA, et al: Dialectical behavior therapy for patients with borderline personality disorder and drug-dependence. Am J Addict 8(4):279–292, 1999 10598211

Linehan MM, Dimeff LA, Reynolds SK, et al: Dialectical behavior therapy versus comprehensive validation therapy plus 12-step for the treatment of opioid dependent women meeting criteria for borderline personality disorder. Drug Alcohol Depend 67(1):13–26, 2002 12062776

Luoma JB, Kohlenberg BS, Hayes SC, Fletcher L: Slow and steady wins the race: a randomized clinical trial of acceptance and commitment therapy targeting shame in substance use disorders. J Consult Clin Psychol 80(1):43–53, 2012 22040285

Marlatt GA, Gordon JR: Relapse Prevention: Maintenance Strategies in the Treatment of Addictive Behaviors. New York, Guilford, 1985

McLellan AT, Lewis DC, O'Brien CP, Kleber HD: Drug dependence, a chronic medical illness: implications for treatment, insurance, and outcomes evaluation. JAMA 284(13):1689–1695, 2000 11015800

Nelson T: Big Wisdom: Little Book; 1,001 Proverbs, Adages, and Precepts to Help You Live a Better Life. Nashville, TN, W Pub Group, 2005

Rösner S, Willutzki R, Zgierska A: Mindfulness-based interventions for substance use disorders. (Protocol). Cochrane Database of Systematic Reviews 2015, Issue 6. Art. No.: CD011723. DOI: 10.1002/14651858.CD011723

Shapiro FR: Who wrote the serenity prayer? Chronicle Review April 28, 2014

Varra AA, Hayes SC, Roget N, Fisher G: A randomized control trial examining the effect of acceptance and commitment training on clinician willingness to use evidence-based pharmacotherapy. J Consult Clin Psychol 76(3):449–458, 2008 18540738

Westbrook C, Creswell JD, Tabibnia G, et al: Mindful attention reduces neural and self-reported cue-induced craving in smokers. Soc Cogn Affect Neurosci 8(1):73–84, 2013 22114078

Whiteford HA, Degenhardt L, Rehm J, et al: Global burden of disease attributable to mental and substance use disorders: findings from the Global Burden of Disease Study 2010. Lancet 382(9904):1575–1586, 2013 23993280

Witkiewitz K, Bowen S, Douglas H, Hsu SH: Mindfulness-based relapse prevention for substance craving. Addict Behav 38(2):1563–1571, 2013 22534451

Zgierska A, Rabago D, Chawla N, et al: Mindfulness meditation for substance use disorders: a systematic review. Subst Abus 30(4):266–294, 2009 19904664

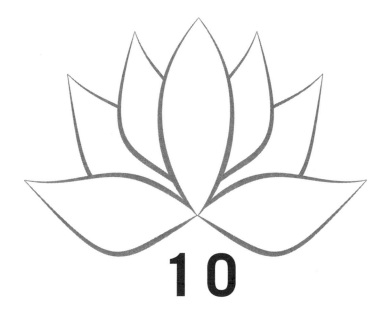

10

Mindful Eating

Kerry Ellen Wangen, M.D., Ph.D.

Let food be thy medicine and medicine be thy food.

Hippocrates

THE Centers for Disease Control and Prevention estimates that 70.7% of the U.S. adult population is now overweight or obese (Centers for Disease Control and Prevention 2013–2014). This epidemic crosses all age groups, income levels, and ethnicities. Despite the prevalence of the problem, there are few treatment options for reducing weight that produce long-term weight loss and are effective and safe. Furthermore, mental health patients have high rates of obesity and often are less able to access obesity treatments because of psychiatric symptoms or other barriers. Contributing to the problem is the fact that many psychiatric medications increase appetite, resulting in weight gain. The addition of binge-eating disorder in DSM-5 (American Psychiatric Association 2013) has increased the attention on the diagnosis and treatment of binge-eating behaviors in the context of binge-eating disorder and bulimia nervosa, as well as in overweight or obese individuals who may not meet diagnostic criteria for an eating disorder. There is a growing need for mental health professionals to intervene and assist patients with weight loss efforts to improve physical health and promote emotional well-being.

Increasing mindfulness toward the experience of eating may help decrease unhealthy eating behaviors, and training in mindful eating offers a safe, relatively low cost, and potentially effective method to help patients decrease binge eating or overeating, lose weight, and maintain a healthier weight. Table 10–1 provides a description of mindful eating. After receiving initial instructions, patients can practice mindful eating at home. While learning the skills, they may find it beneficial to have concurrent support and help with problem solving from a trained mindfulness practitioner. Because mindful eating practices are safe, they can be offered to children and teens with minimal risk, and because eating patterns from early life frequently persist into adulthood, mindful eating has the potential to benefit individuals throughout life.

In this chapter, we review the origin of mindful eating practices, the possible mechanisms of action for how mindfulness may alter eating behavior, clinical methods to implement mindful eating, research on the use of mindful eating, and instructions on how professionals can train patients in mindful eating in a variety of clinical settings even during a single clinical encounter.

TABLE 10–1. Mindful eating practices

Avoiding any other activity (e.g., talking, reading, watching TV, driving) while eating

Slowing the pace of eating

Being aware of

    Physical sensations (e.g., taste, hunger, fullness)

    Thoughts (e.g., craving, like or dislike, critical inner comments)

    Emotions (e.g., anxiety, excitement, joy, numbness)

Maintaining full awareness of and attention to the sight, smell, taste, and texture of food

Staying with a moment-to-moment experience of eating and coming back to the eating experience when the mind naturally drifts away

Bringing curiosity and interest, without judgment, to what is happening inside one's body while engaging in eating

Being conscious of the periods before and after eating

History of Mindful Eating Practice

Mindful eating practices were first introduced in the U.S. mainstream in the book *Full Catastrophe Living* by Jon Kabat-Zinn (1990). He went on to develop Mindfulness-Based Stress Reduction (MBSR), which is one of the treatments used in research studies on mindfulness, including mindful eating studies. The practice of applying mindfulness to the process of eating has its roots in Buddhist teachings and has been practiced for centuries. The Buddhist practices and the origins of bringing mindfulness to eating are described in the book *Savor: Mindful Eating, Mindful Life* (Nhat Hanh and Cheung 2010). Mindful eating practices available in the Western world focus on how to be more in tune with appetite, the process of eating, the needs of the body, and the thoughts and actions that may hinder the ability to make positive changes in eating behaviors.

How Mindfulness May Influence Eating Behaviors

Overeating can be caused by a wide range of factors. Individuals may overeat for psychological reasons or in response to physical sensations, social influences, habit patterns, or external environmental cues. There are psychological processes that precede or lead to the onset of eating, such as hunger, craving, previous hedonic responses to food, motivation to eat or not eat, or an anticipated reward from eating. There are additional processes that relate to cessation of eating, or avoidance of eating, including fullness, external cues, or a feeling of satisfaction (French et al. 2012). Mindful eating practices can influence when a person starts and stops eating and when the person chooses to eat or not eat. Engaging in mindfulness before, during, and after eating can help patients better match their food intake to their bodies' needs and avoid negative behaviors such as overeating, eating foods that are not supportive of their health, and binge eating.

Psychosomatic theories of overeating suggest that some individuals have a reduced ability to distinguish between physical hunger and emotional arousal and thus may be prone to overeating or pathological eating behaviors. Emotional eating can occur consciously or unconsciously when an individual consumes food or beverages to reduce an undesired emotion, such as anxiety or sadness, or to produce a desired emotion, such as joy or connection with others. Eating based on emotions is not necessarily pathological, but in the extreme it can lead to disordered eating behaviors or chronic overeating. Mindful eating can provide a method to inquire within to sort out physical sensations and emotional states prior to eating and during eating, thereby providing the individual with information that can alter eating behavior.

Dysregulation theories suggest that some individuals have poor recognition of hunger and satiety cues. This lack of recognition may preexist overeating or binge eating and may be a consequence of chronic lack of attention to these cues. Mindful eating may enhance a person's recognition of satiety and hunger cues, leading to improved restraint in food intake. Eating mindfully can slow the eating process and increase the length of time for satiety signaling by gastrointestinal hormones, such as glucagon-like peptide, cholecystokinin, and peptide YY. Mindfulness also creates more awareness of the physical sensations, such as abdominal distention or loss of hunger. The observation of these sensations provides information to the individual, who then has the opportunity to alter the total amount of food, pace of eating, or types of food consumed. Instead of eating to the point of physical fullness, individuals can adjust to stop eating when their hunger is satisfied rather than when they become full. This recognition of satiety can lead to a reduction in food intake if individuals notice they are getting full and consciously choose to stop eating. Individuals may also become more aware of foods that cause undesirable effects, such as reflux or abdominal pain, and make adjustments in the types of foods they consume at future meals.

The *externality theory* suggests that some individuals may have heightened sensitivity to external food cues. This increased sensitivity to the sight, smell, or discussion of food can lead to negative eating behaviors, such as eating when one is not physically hungry, the inability to avoid a food that is not healthy, or overeating. In the United States, food is easily available in many settings beyond grocery stores and restaurants, including from vending machines, check-out counters in many shops, fast food outlets, convenience stores, gas stations, and street vendors' carts. This increased visibility of food can pose a challenge to individuals who react to the sight of foods even when they are not hungry. Individuals with high levels of impulsivity may engage in eating far more often than needed because of the high visibility of food. Learning mindful eating may help individuals gain improved restraint in situations where eating is driven by external cues. Improved restraint can lead to an increased feeling of control over problematic eating behaviors and enhance emotional, psychological, and physical well-being.

Mindful eating provides a wealth of information to individuals about their eating behaviors, including psychological, physical, and external triggers of undesired eating. They become aware of their thoughts before, during, and after eating, thus gaining insights into negative patterns of eating; they can then process these insights with the hope of overcoming eating behaviors that are causing distress or having negative impacts on health. Developing an awareness of both why they are eating and how overeating or pathological eating behaviors are occurring in their daily life can lead individuals to change their eating behaviors.

These insights are likely to be enhanced through support and discussion with a mental health professional trained in mindfulness. The professional can help an individual to fully process the origins of the thoughts and motivations, as well as support the planning and monitoring of beneficial behavior changes. For example, traumatic experiences in life, including negative experiences related to eating, lack of access to food, or being bullied for body shape or size, can influence present-day eating patterns and thoughts about food and body. Gaining insight into these associations through mindful eating, as well as having support from a mental health provider, may help patients change eating behaviors through processing these past experiences.

Mindful eating interventions can be tailored to psychological, physical, and behavioral causes of overeating that can lead to binge eating, overweight, or obesity. Mindful eating may help individuals to be aware of thoughts and experiences that lead to overeating, binge eating, or the inability to stay on an eating plan that is designed to improve physical health through weight loss or changes such as improving glycemic control. Mindfulness can enhance a person's ability to restrain or reduce food intake to healthy levels. A mental health professional can provide the person with assistance in processing these insights and developing a plan to make beneficial changes. Support groups may also offer an opportunity to enhance skill development in adopting and maintaining a mindful eating practice.

Current Protocols for Teaching Mindful Eating

A variety of studies have examined various forms of teaching mindful eating and the outcomes in different patient populations, with varying degrees of suc- cess. Study populations have included individuals with diagnosed eating disor- ders, individuals with binge-eating episodes with or without an eating disorder diagnosis, obese individuals, potential bariatric surgery patients, individuals with type 2 diabetes, and other groups. The studies have taught mindful eating within the context of general mindfulness training in group sessions. The amount of mindfulness training, and specifically the focus on mindful eating, has varied widely. Some of the therapies used also contained other components of mindfulness, such as distress tolerance and acceptance skills.

The therapies used most often in mindful eating research to date include MBSR, acceptance and commitment therapy (ACT), dialectical behavior ther- apy (DBT), Mindfulness-Based Cognitive Therapy (MBCT), and Mindfulness- Based Eating Awareness Training (MB-EAT). MB-EAT, which is less well known than the other therapies, was adapted from MBSR by Kristeller et al. (2014). Every MB-EAT session is focused on developing mindfulness skills; patients participate in weekly exercises on mindful eating, home practice of mindful eating, and daily practice of mindfulness meditations. MBSR, ACT, DBT, and MBCT focus primarily on developing general mindfulness skills and do not tend to have a significant focus on mindful eating in particular. Studies done to date have varied in the amount of mindfulness, specifically the focus on mindful eating, in sessions and the practice requirements between sessions in research and clinical settings.

Mindful Eating Research

There is a rapidly expanding body of research in mindful eating that has been done in a variety of patient populations, including healthy college students, overweight adults, and patients with eating disorders. The methods for training subjects in mindful eating vary widely.

A systematic review by Wanden-Berghe et al. (2011) included eight studies conducted in patients with diagnosed eating disorders, including anorexia ner- vosa, bulimia nervosa, and binge-eating disorder. The studies used general mindfulness interventions or cognitive-behavioral-type mindfulness protocols, including MBCT, DBT, and ACT. The reviewers concluded, on the basis of the positive outcomes observed in these eight studies, that mindfulness-based therapies may be effective in the treatment of eating disorders. The outcomes differed across studies, which included endpoints such as reduction in binge eating or emotional eating, changes in attitudes toward eating, and more awareness of hunger and satiety.

In a literature review, O'Reilly et al. (2014) looked at the effectiveness of mindfulness-based interventions for different obesity-related behaviors, including binge eating, emotional eating, and external eating. *External eating* has been described as eating in response to any external food-related cues, including the smell, sight, or discussion of a food. The 21 studies used a wide variety of methods for implementing mindfulness training through combined mindfulness and cognitive-behavioral therapies, including MBCT, MBSR, and ACT. The results showed that mindfulness-based interventions led to improvement in obesity-related behaviors in 86% of the reviewed studies, with moderate to large effect sizes. The behaviors showing the most improvement included binge eating, emotional eating, and external eating. In 9 of the 10 studies that reported weight, the interventions had a positive impact on body weight outcomes, but effect sizes for body weight changes were small.

In a systematic review, Katterman et al. (2014) examined the impact of mindfulness meditation on overeating behaviors, including binge eating, emotional eating, and weight loss. Fourteen articles were included in their review, and subjects were from a variety of populations including, among others, postoperative bariatric surgery patients who binge eat, patients in treatment for type 2 diabetes, and patients presenting for stress reduction or treatment of stress eating. The amount and type of mindfulness training in the studies varied widely. The reviewers concluded that mindfulness interventions effectively reduced binge eating and emotional overeating behaviors for those individuals who engaged in these behaviors at baseline. The postintervention changes in weight were small or nonsignificant, with the positive changes seen in those studies in which weight loss was a primary outcome.

A systematic review and meta-analysis by Godfrey et al. (2015) examined studies on mindfulness-based interventions for individuals with binge-eating behavior, with or without a diagnosis of binge-eating disorder. Nineteen studies were included in the analysis. The interventions used a variety of methods to train subjects in mindfulness, including MBCT, DBT, ACT, MB-EAT, MBSR, and adaptations of these. They found medium-large and large effect sizes for these interventions on reduction of binge eating. The reviewers concluded that mindfulness-based interventions can be considered effective for binge eating.

Additional studies have been done since the above-mentioned reviews were completed. Ouwens et al. (2015) examined the association between mindfulness and eating behavior styles, including restrained, emotional, and external eating, in 335 obese men and women who were candidates for bariatric surgery. Mindfulness was found to be associated with more restrained eating behaviors and with fewer emotional and externally cued eating behaviors in this population. Mason et al. (2016) examined the impact of a mindfulness-based intervention on mindful eating, sweets consumption, and fasting glucose in 194 obese adults participating in a Stroke Hyperglycemia Insulin Network Effort (SHINE) trial. The subjects participated in a 5.5-month diet and exercise program with or without mindfulness training using MB-EAT. Those subjects who did not receive mindfulness training were taught cognitive-behavioral and relaxation tools for stress reduction. Increases in mindful eating were associated with decreased consumption of sweets and lower fasting glucose. The mindfulness group had increased mindful eating and maintained baseline fasting glucose at 12 months, whereas the active control group had increased fasting glucose over this same period.

One challenge in the interpretation of the research to date is that studies have used a wide variety of methods to train subjects in mindful eating. The different protocols also vary significantly in the amount of instruction in mindful eating, ranging from a single session to weekly reinforcement of mindful eating during the study intervention period. The studies also vary in the amount of focus given to building general mindfulness skills. Some research has used mindfulness-based interventions that are unique, but the majority of studies have used established therapies, such as MBSR, MBCT, DBT, or ACT, which have a mindfulness-based component that is then applied to eating in a single or multiple sessions during the intervention. These established therapies also contain other elements, such as the development of distress tolerance and acceptance skills. Research to date has not demonstrated what methods of teaching mindful eating may be most effective, how many sessions are needed, what differences exist between patient populations, or what measures are best for assessing mindful eating or eating behaviors.

Future research is needed to sort out which elements of the various forms of mindfulness training have the greatest impact on undesired eating behaviors and positive weight change. There is a need for continued research with different patient groups, including those with diagnosed eating disorders, as well as those who do not meet criteria for an eating disorder but are engaging in eating behaviors that have negative impacts on their emotional or physical well-being. Different protocols may vary in their effectiveness in different groups and on the key endpoints of interest in these populations. Further studies are needed to shed light on how best to translate findings to the clinical setting. Despite the preliminary nature of the current body of evidence for mindful eating training, findings suggest that mindful eating has great potential to alter undesired eating behaviors, especially binge eating. However, the research to date does not indicate a robust impact on weight reduction. The mindful eating training may need to be expanded in the protocols to have more mindful eating practice in-group sessions, as well as more between-session development of the skills with daily home practice, such as that used in MB-EAT. Given that eating, or not eating, is influenced by social, emotional, physical, and external cues, patients may need some level of individual attention by professionals to assist in problem solving. Mindful eating skills may also be more effective in some patient groups when combined with other methods, such as nutritional education, individual therapy, and weight management skills.

Incorporating Mindful Eating in Clinical Practice

Research trials on mindful eating to date have focused on group interventions. The group setting provides a cost-effective way to provide the intervention and offers an environment in which individuals can learn from one another, fostering support among members and thereby enhancing therapeutic connections between individuals. Depending on what is available locally, patients may be referred to group therapies using MBSR, MBCT, ACT, or DBT.

A patient can learn mindful eating techniques in individual sessions with a provider trained in mindfulness practices, specifically mindful eating, and then the patient's out-of-session practice of the skills can be reinforced in follow-up sessions. Individual sessions also offer the patient the opportunity to work through barriers, such as previous trauma or strong emotions that arise during mindfulness practice, that a patient may be reluctant to share in a group setting or that may cause resistance to adopting the practice of mindful eating. On the basis of research to date, individuals who have challenges with negative eating behaviors or who are overweight vary widely in their genetics, previous environmental exposures, and current food behaviors. By targeting mindful eating intervention and practice to individuals' specific needs, clinicians may help patients work through their individual difficulties with emotional eating, impulsivity, or sensitivity to environmental food cues. Individual sessions provide further opportunity to personalize the mindful eating practices to target patients' challenging thoughts or other barriers that hinder the reduction of undesired food behaviors.

One basic form of mindfulness instruction that is particularly useful for eating issues is a technique called RAIN, an acronym for the steps of the process: **R**ecognize, **A**ccept/allow, **I**nvestigate, **N**onjudgment. RAIN is offered by *vipassanā* teachers at centers such as the Insight Meditation Society Retreat Center and Spirit Rock Meditation Center (for locations and Web sites, see "Retreat Centers Offering Mindfulness-Based Programs" in Appendix B, "Mindfulness Resources"). Figure 10–1 lists the elements of RAIN, a four-step process that is easy to remember, often yields insights, and assists in the processing and acceptance of the immediate experience.

Recognize	• Notice the physical sensations, thoughts, or emotions occurring in the present moment.

Accept/allow	• Let the sensations, thoughts, or emotions be present without trying to change anything or pushing them away.

Investigate	• Explore the sensations, thoughts, or emotions arising with curiosity and interest. How do they change with attention and time?

Nonjudgment	• Drop any criticism or judgments that arise and stay with the moment-to-moment experience.

FIGURE 10–1. Elements of RAIN, a form of mindfulness instruction that is useful for eating issues.

Source. Adapted from Brach 2013.

Even if the focus of a patient's therapy is not on mindfulness or eating behaviors, a simple introduction to mindfulness practice provides a rich learning opportunity and may inspire patients to want to learn more about mindfulness. A mindful eating exercise can be used in a resident lecture, therapy group, patient education class, or other setting to give individuals an introduction to mindfulness and specifically to mindful eating. People report it is a rich and eye opening experience to place so much attention on the eating experience. The typical introductory exercise uses a grape or a raisin, but one can also use another natural food item. A sample script for the mindful eating exercise is provided on p. 158. It is important to go very slowly through this mindful eating exercise, perhaps spending 8–10 minutes total for the eating process. Participant insights come from the silence and the time to observe all sensations and thoughts that arise during the eating process. If more time is available, it can be helpful to allow a few minutes for participants to write down some details of their experience, including their thoughts and feelings about the exercise and any emotions that came up during the experience.

Sample script for mindful eating

Place the grape so it is close at hand.

Close your eyes and take a few slow deep breaths, allowing your whole belly to expand on each inhalation, and on each exhalation allow any tension or stress to release with the out breath.

Move your awareness into your feet, then your legs, your torso, and into your arms and hands. Feel your whole body sitting here in the chair, and just allow any tension to let go with each out breath.

Now bring your awareness to your mouth. Note any tastes or sensations present. Is your mouth starting to water in anticipation of the grape?

Without chewing, place the grape in your mouth, and close your eyes again.

What do you notice first?

Explore the shape, the texture, and note any flavors before chewing.

Where on your tongue are the flavors most intense?

Now use your teeth to bite the grape one time. How does this change the experience?

What thoughts are going through your mind right now?

When you are ready, slowly and completely chew the grape.

Try to chew it at least 15 times.

When you are ready to swallow, do so and pay close attention to the sensations.

How do you feel in this moment? Is there desire for another grape?

How is this intense focus on eating different from how you usually eat?

What would it be like to eat an entire meal with this level of mindfulness?

When you are ready, open your eyes.

This mindful eating exercise with a grape (or other natural food item) is enhanced when it is immediately repeated with a highly sweetened processed fruit-flavored chewy candy (e.g., Starburst or Skittles) to contrast natural and processed sugars, as well as natural versus artificial flavors. This comparison surprises people with how unpleasant or intense a highly processed, refined sweetener tastes compared with natural fruit sugar. People have reported that placing so much attention on the eating experience is a rich and eye-opening experience.

Many resources are available to support independent learning about and application of mindful eating outside of an individual or group therapy intervention. The Center for Mindful Eating Web site (http://thecenterformindfuleating.org) includes guidelines, webinars, handouts, and other kinds of information. Several books are also very helpful:

- *Eating Mindfully: How to End Mindless Eating and Enjoy a Balanced Relationship With Food* (2012, New Harbinger) and the workbook *Eat, Drink and Be Mindful: How to End Your Struggle With Mindless Eating and Start Savoring Food With Intention and Joy* (2008, New Harbinger) by Susan Albers
- *Savor: Mindful Eating, Mindful Life* by Thich Nhat Hanh and Lilian Cheung (2010, Harper Collins)
- *Mindful Eating: A Guide to Rediscovering a Healthy and Joyful Relationship With Food* by Jan Chozen Bays (2009, Shambala)

Challenges in Implementing a Mindful Eating Practice

There are several common obstacles in teaching and practicing mindful eating that are important to highlight. First, patients may not have access to mindful eating groups or trained individual providers locally, or they may lack financial resources to pay for these services. Books and Web sites offer information that may help clinicians and patients get started in these practices.

Second, when individuals are using food and eating as a way to cope with life stressors or strong emotions, they may meet the practice of mindful eating with resistance, or they may become overwhelmed with the emotional content or life stressors they had been suppressing through eating behaviors. Such an individual may need to work with a mental health provider to enhance the patient's range of coping skills, as well as the processing of emotional content, so that he or she can fully engage in mindful eating without becoming sabotaged by other factors.

Finally, most people find that learning and implementing behavior change is challenging. Motivational interviewing can be helpful to assess an individual's readiness for change. Providing a supportive, nonjudgmental atmosphere and a flexible plan for mindful eating can help individuals find the best approach for their own needs and goals. It is critical to set specific, measurable, and attainable goals for implementing mindful eating practices successfully.

Mindfulness develops with practice, so setting a goal of bringing mindfulness to the first portion of a meal or to one meal per week may be a good starting point. Some individuals may want to set a goal such as not eating while driving or watching TV, or maybe eating in silence for some meals each week. As a person's mindful eating skills develop, the goals can be increased. It is essential to reduce the potential for self-judgment or inner criticism that can lead to resistance to mindful eating. Setting a realistic goal for weekly practice will enhance the individual's success in implementing mindful eating.

Key Points for Further Study and Reflection

- The application of mindfulness to eating behavior has the potential to reduce negative eating behaviors in individuals with eating disorders, binge-eating behaviors, or obesity.
- Mindful eating may help individuals reach or maintain a healthy weight and support a positive relationship with food and eating.
- Mindful eating practice enhances an individual's awareness of physical, emotional, and psychological factors that affect eating or overeating and provides the skills to change current patterns of intake to enhance health and well-being.
- Mindful eating is likely to be more effective when individuals are also practicing mindfulness in the rest of their daily life, because they will have greater development of mindfulness skills.
- The development of mindful eating skills, as well as the successful implementation of these skills, is likely enhanced when working with a mental health provider who has had mindfulness training.

References

American Psychiatric Association: Diagnostic and Statistical Manual of Mental Disorders, 5th Edition. Arlington, VA, American Psychiatric Association, 2013
Brach T: True Refuge: Finding Peace and Freedom in Your Own Awakened Heart. New York, Random House, 2013

Centers for Disease Control and Prevention: CDC National Center for Health Statistics, 2013/2014. Available at: www.cdc.gov/nchs/fastats/obesity-overweight.htm. Accessed June 20, 2016.

French SA, Epstein LH, Jeffery RW, et al: Eating behavior dimensions: associations with energy intake and body weight. A review. Appetite 59(2):541–549, 2012 22796186

Godfrey KM, Gallo LC, Afari N: Mindfulness-based interventions for binge eating: a systematic review and meta-analysis. J Behav Med 38(2):348–362, 2015 25417199

Kabat-Zinn J: Full Catastrophe Living: Using the Wisdom of Your Body and Mind to Face Stress, Pain, and Illness. New York, Delacorte, 1990

Katterman SN, Kleinman BM, Hood MM, et al: Mindfulness meditation as an intervention for binge eating, emotional eating, and weight loss: a systematic review. Eat Behav 15(2):197–204, 2014 24854804

Kristeller J, Wolever RQ, Sheets V: Mindfulness-based eating awareness training (MB-EAT) for binge eating: a randomized clinical trial. Mindfulness 5(3):282–297, 2014

Mason AE, Epel ES, Kristeller J, et al: Effects of a mindfulness-based intervention on mindful eating, sweets consumption, and fasting glucose levels in obese adults: data from the SHINE randomized controlled trial. J Behav Med 39(2):201–213, 2016 26563148

Nhat Hanh TN, Cheung L: Savor: Mindful Eating, Mindful Life. New York, HarperCollins, 2010

O'Reilly GA, Cook L, Spruijt-Metz D, Black DS: Mindfulness-based interventions for obesity-related eating behaviours: a literature review. Obes Rev 15(6):453–461, 2014 24636206

Ouwens MA, Schiffer AA, Visser LI, et al: Mindfulness and eating behaviour styles in morbidly obese males and females. Appetite 87:62–67, 2015 25478687

Wanden-Berghe RG, Sanz-Valero J, Wanden-Berghe C: The application of mindfulness to eating disorders treatment: a systematic review. Eat Disord 19(1):34–48, 2011 21181578

11

Mindfulness and Technology

Matthew Diamond, M.D., Ph.D.
Patricia Zheng, M.D.
Sarah Zoogman, Ph.D.

If you just sit and observe, you will see how restless your mind is.... [O]ver time it does calm, and when it does...that's when your intuition starts to blossom and you start to see things more clearly.... [Y]ou see a tremendous expanse in the moment. You see so much more than you could see before.

Steve Jobs (quoted by Isaacson 2015)

TECHNOLOGY HAS FORGED the framework of modern society and enabled the increased life expectancy and comforts associated with contemporary living. Recent advances have created exponential growth in the sharing and processing of information, and the rapid adoption of mobile technology has dramatically changed how we interact with each other and our environment. As a result, most of us spend a large portion of our waking hours engaged with device screens, and we perform much of our communication through electronic media.

Although modern technology has many benefits and has increased our overall productivity, its use (and especially its misuse) has the potential to distract us from the present moment and decrease awareness of our inner experience and immediate surroundings. These effects explicitly compromise our mindfulness. Although technology can hinder our mindfulness, it can also be used to enhance mindfulness. And mindfulness can be used as a tool to mediate our interactions with technology.

In this chapter we focus on Internet-based and mobile technologies, exemplified by the smartphone, and address the following questions: 1) How can mindfulness be used to inform our relationship with technology? 2) In what ways can technology be used to promote mindfulness? 3) Can mindfulness be used to foster technological innovation? We touch on the nascent research in this emerging field and provide a practical guide for using mindfulness to mediate one's relationship with technology. We also present examples of mindfulness-related devices and applications, with the understanding that the rapid pace of technological innovation may make some of the items discussed obsolete.

Using Everyday Technology Mindfully

In 2014, the average American adult spent more than 11 waking hours per day engaged with electronic media, mostly through screens (Nielsen 2015). Children ages 8–18 years spend on average more than 50 hours per week using media outside of school (Rideout et al. 2010). Seventy-three percent of teenagers own smartphones, and 24% of teenagers report going online "almost constantly," with girls dominating social media and boys devoting more time to video gaming (Lenhart 2015). Teenagers report using text messaging more than face-to-face socialization (Lenhart 2012).

The possible negative effects caused by excessive use of the Internet, especially among youth, have been well documented (Lam 2014; Moreno et al. 2011; Strasburger et al. 2010), and some arguments have been made that Internet addiction disorder should be added to DSM (Block 2008). The American Academy of Pediatrics recently reported that "excessive media use can lead to attention problems, school difficulties, sleep and eating disorders, and obesity" (American Academy of Pediatrics 2015). There is a growing concern that youths' face-to-face communication skills, including the ability to read facial expressions, and their emotional intelligence and intuition, may be negatively affected by excessive electronic media use (Giedd 2012). Despite the dangers of inappropriate and excessive Internet use, it is worth acknowledging the benefits that modern technology has brought to education and the innovative opportunities that digital media offers (Higgins et al. 2012).

Given the central role that modern technology plays in our lives, it is important to consider how we can use technology mindfully. At meditation centers such as Spirit Rock in Woodacre, California, where courses and retreats are offered year round, participants are instructed to refrain from phone and Internet use. Taking a break from mobile technology and the Internet has many benefits, including the ability to gain insight into our relationship with modern technology in its absence. Indeed, there is some evidence that spending punctuated periods of time in a natural setting with limited technology can mitigate some of the effects of media overconsumption (Uhls et al. 2014). Rather than focus on these "technology-fasting" interventions, however, in this chapter we focus on strategies to use technology wisely in our hyperconnected native environment. The challenge here lies in using technology as an opportunity for mindful living rather than a distraction from it.

We as clinicians need to assess whether and how our own use of technology may be unhealthy. Each of us should pause and ask ourselves: How often do I use a smartphone, computer, or the Internet? How frequently do I check e-mail? Do my interactions with these technologies set the tone of my autonomic nervous system, emotional state, or activities for the day? Does a lack of access to my everyday technologies cause me significant distress? The answers to these questions may provide insight into our dependence on these modern technologies and inspire us to shift our relationship with them.

For decades the Vietnamese Buddhist monk and mindfulness proponent Thich Nhat Hanh has taught how to take a mindful stance in everyday interactions with technology. He has compared modern technology to a knife, in that it can be used to nourish (e.g., prepare food to feed one's family) or to destroy. In order to use technology to nourish, he advises bringing compassion and insight to one's interactions with technology (Nhat Hanh 2013).

The manner in which we can bring mindfulness to our interactions with technology can be categorized in two ways (with some overlap between the two): 1) reframing our relationship with technological objects through an attitudinal shift and 2) using specific awareness-promoting features of the technology. The reader is invited to apply these approaches to his or her moment-to-moment interactions with everyday technology; below are examples of this application with some of our most commonly used objects.

Clock

Perceived lack of time is a significant source of stress in today's society (Gebel 2012). The default way to relate to looking at a clock and checking the time seems to be with stress and anxiety (e.g., "I can't believe it's already so late"; "Where did the time go?") and mindlessness. Through a shift in awareness, however, a clock can actually facilitate mindfulness. Checking the time can become a conscious act, the clock serving as a reminder to breathe in and out; notice thoughts, feelings, and body sensations that are occurring; and bring awareness to the present moment.

To facilitate a reframing of our relationship with the clock, we can use its built-in features for the promotion of mindfulness. In Plum Village, Nhat Hanh's retreat center in the south of France, there are grandfather clocks in the communal indoor spaces that sound bells every 15 minutes during the day. Whenever the bells sound, people are invited to pause what they are doing, breathe, and return to the present moment. From the authors' experience, it is a magical moment.

Most people have access to a timer or alarm that they can use specifically to bring awareness to the present moment, and hardware and software that can activate periodic "mindfulness bells" are now available. Wearable devices with internal clocks and sensors can also be used to help reframe people's relationship with time (see the section "Technology for Promoting Mindfulness" later in this chapter).

Phone

Like the clock, the phone can be a source of stress, anxiety, and mindlessness, but if we can shift our relationship with our phone, we can use it to promote mindfulness and well-being for ourselves and others. Even before cellular phones began to dominate our cultural landscape, Nhat Hanh was teaching how to bring mindful awareness to using the telephone. He advises not picking up the phone on the first ring but rather using that first ring as a reminder to stop talking or thinking, enjoy breathing in and out, and smile. On the second ring of the phone, he recommends taking another breath and enjoying the moment. He does not worry about callers hanging up, he says, because if they have something really important to say, he knows they will not hang up so soon. On the third ring, he suggests standing up and walking to the phone calmly and mindfully, breathing and smiling, with dignity. The calmness and concentration nurtured through this awareness will be reflected in the sound of one's voice and in what one says (Nhat Hanh 2014).

Today, with 90% of American adults owning cell phones, the majority owning smartphones, and most smartphone users keeping their phones with them for most hours of the day and night (Smith 2015), using phones mindfully is increasingly important. Because smartphones serve not only as tools for communication but also as timekeeping devices and major conduits for e-mail, Web browsing, and digital media, they carry a responsibility for their use that combines the issues addressed in this subsection, those in the previous subsection for clocks, and in the next subsection for the Internet.

Limiting smartphone use at bedtime and during meals is often recommended as a first step toward its mindful use. One can use the built-in features that smartphones already contain, such as the "do not disturb" mode, which allows users to send all or most calls to voicemail. A variety of smartphone applications (apps) specifically designed to promote mindfulness are discussed later in this chapter (see the section "Technology for Promoting Mindfulness").

Internet

It has been well documented that the Internet and e-mail, along with cell phones, have increased the number of people we interact with regularly, our overall productivity, and the flexibility of our work hours (Purcell and Rainie 2014). More than 30% of American workers, however, feel that these technologies have caused them to work an increased number of total hours per week (Purcell and Rainie 2014), and the ability to work outside of the office, including on weekends and evenings, can disrupt traditional boundaries between work and home life. In addition, surfing the Web can easily become a distracted and mindless activity, consuming lots of time without providing nourishment.

A number of special tools are available to monitor how much time we spend on the computer and to increase mindfulness of what we are pursuing online. Apps such as RescueTime, which runs securely in the background, allow the user to create goals (e.g., spend only 1 hour per day on e-mail), to receive notifications if too much time is spent on an activity, and to block distracting Web sites. Specialized tools such as these provide a way for individuals to gain awareness about their own use of technology. However, making a simple commitment to certain habits, such as not checking one's e-mail in the middle of the night even if awake, may be a useful way for health practitioners and patients alike to redefine their relationship with the Internet.

Car

The automobile is not traditionally categorized as mobile technology, but its inclusion in this chapter is merited by its everyday utility, its emerging participation in the Internet of Things (see the section "Future Directions of Mindful Technology" later in this chapter), and the way its use is explicitly influenced by smartphones and other devices. Mindfulness teacher Sylvia Boorstein (2006) describes how to bring compassion and awareness to driving. Consider how often we drive on automatic pilot, being out of touch with the present moment, and arrive feeling that we have lost the time we were in the car; how often the experience of driving (e.g., sitting in traffic, dealing with other drivers) causes unpleasant emotional states (e.g., frustration, anger, rage) that stay with us even after we have arrived at our destination; or how often we engage in distractions (e.g., texting) while driving, losing sight of the dangers of these behaviors for both ourselves and others.

Although frequently used mindlessly, the car can be used as a tool for becoming more present. In fact, the experience of driving can be used to more deeply appreciate the interconnectedness and interdependence of all beings. On the highway, each driver is dependent on every other driver to stay in his or her lane so that everybody arrives safely at his or her destination (Boorstein 2006). Nhat Hanh (2006) composed a special *gatha*, or meditative verse, for driving:

> Before starting the car
> I know where I'm going.
> The car and I are one.
> If the car goes fast, I go fast.
> If the car goes slowly, I go slowly. (p. 72)

Verses like these can be used as tools to bring intentionality and awareness to our daily use of technology.

Just as one can bring mindfulness to driving a car, one can also make a mindful choice about whether to use a car at all. Indeed, a movement to embrace slower modes of transportation, such as walking and biking, has been viewed as a way to cultivate mindful awareness and transcend the everyday through spatial practice (Osbaldiston 2013).

Technology for Promoting Mindfulness

Not only does our use of technology benefit from a mindful approach, but technology itself is providing tools to nurture and promote mindfulness in a number of ways. First, in the same manner that technology has increased our access to all information, it can connect us with an online community of mindfulness resources. Second, specialized software, particularly mobile apps, has been developed to facilitate a mindful practice. Third, a number of smart connected devices have begun to emerge to support mindful living as part of the nascent Internet of Things, discussed in the section "Future Directions of Mindful Technology." (See Table

11–1 at the end of the chapter for descriptions of representative technological tools for promoting mindfulness and links to more information about those tools.)

Technology Facilitating Access to Mindfulness Resources

There has been a proliferation of online resources on mindfulness. Searching YouTube videos using the term *mindfulness* brings up more than 400,000 results. These include talks by Jon Kabat-Zinn on the research supporting mindfulness practice and by Thich Nhat Hanh on the basics of mindfulness practice. Through the Internet one can quickly and easily obtain outstanding mindfulness books, including those by Buddhist Nun Pema Chodron (e.g., *When Things Fall Apart* and *The Places That Scare You*) and *vipassanā* teacher Jack Kornfield (e.g., *A Path With Heart* and *After the Ecstasy, The Laundry*). In addition to videos and books, the Internet offers information about local in-person classes and online mindfulness courses. Online courses include Mindfulness-Based Stress Reduction (MBSR), an 8-week course developed by Kabat-Zinn, which is composed of a variety of formal mindfulness practices, including mindful movement and sitting meditation (Khoury et al. 2013). The University of California, Los Angeles offers an interactive online course that includes lectures, practice, and discussion, as well as online meditations (UCLA Mindful Awareness Research Center 2015). Technology also allows people interested in mindfulness to connect through social Web sites.

Mobile Applications Supporting Mindfulness

A growing number of mobile apps support practicing mindfulness. These apps function in numerous ways, including 1) bringing our awareness to the present moment; 2) increasing awareness of our inner experience, mood, and surroundings; 3) providing feedback and direction (e.g., "your breath is rapid; take 10 deep mindful breaths"); and 4) helping us to appreciate our interconnectedness.

Mobile mindfulness apps have the ability to support the user in bringing mindfulness practice into everyday life by promoting mindfulness practice on the go. Headspace, an app marketed as a "gym membership for the mind," has modules that teach meditation basics and that provide guided meditation focusing on specific areas of interest (e.g., relationships, stress) and everyday activities (e.g., cooking). It tracks the user's progress and offers the opportunity to connect with friends to motivate one another. Cofounded by Andy Puddicombe, a former Buddhist monk, Headspace boasted 2 million users in 2015. Buddhify, another mindfulness-based mobile app, allows users to choose a meditation that corresponds to what they are doing (e.g., going to sleep, eating) to support incorporating mindfulness into their daily activities; it also allows users to track their progress. A crowdsource app called mSpot allows users to upload and suggest off-the-beaten-path public spaces, including gardens, parks, churches, and beaches, that are ideal for meditation. Another app, 7 Second Meditation, allows users to set timed reminders and push notifications to breathe, to reflect on life, or to be present.

Although there is much evidence to support mindfulness meditation in the treatment of a variety of disorders, including anxiety, depression, and stress (Khoury et al. 2013), there is limited evidence to support the therapeutic benefits of mindfulness apps (Plaza et al. 2013). Some of the limited data available on the efficacy of these tools come from studies of stress (Carissoli et al. 2015), smoking cessation (Davis et al. 2015), and overall wellness (Howells et al. 2014). A recent review of mindfulness apps highlights that further research is needed on their efficacy, and further refinement of apps is needed to enhance the user experience (Mani et al. 2015).

Mindfulness-Related Devices

Devices designed to promote a mindful lifestyle are increasing in number. Some of these devices simply provide reminders throughout the day. Others contain sensors that aim to detect the user's behavior or physiological state and provide feedback and direction. Still others attempt to modify the user's environment to make it more conducive to being mindful.

The Meaning to Pause wristband vibrates every 60–90 minutes to remind the user to return to the present moment. There are also wearable devices, such as the Fitbit Flex and Misfit Shine 2 fitness and sleep monitors, that provide an alert if the user is sedentary for more than a specific period of time. These reminders for users to avoid prolonged sedentary behavior can be viewed as "bells of mindfulness" about one's physical activity throughout the day. In fact, one could argue that the greatest impact of wearable fitness monitors comes from increased mindfulness about the user's activity, sleep, and overall health. Prana and Spire are wearable devices specifically devoted to stress; they contain sensors that track breathing and other parameters to help recognize stress, and then provide biofeedback as part of a mindfulness practice. Muse is a headband-like wearable device that claims to monitor its user's emotional state while providing feedback via a mobile app to facilitate meditation. Thync, another wearable device for the forehead, uses low-energy waveforms purportedly to stimulate the brain and induce emotional states of calm and excitation. Somadome is a personal meditation pod that combines color immersion therapy and audiotherapy with the goal of increasing productivity, mental acuity, focus, and overall well-being and employee retention.

There is currently a paucity of validation studies on devices that promote mindfulness (Yu et al. 2012), and this is especially true of consumer mindfulness tools. Further validation studies are warranted.

Future Directions of Mindful Technology

There is growing recognition that in a technologically hyperconnected environment, nurturing mindfulness in the workplace is important for employees to be innovative and productive, as well as to feel satisfied and healthy. This movement to bring mindfulness into corporate America has been spearheaded by the leading technology companies of Silicon Valley. Google, for example, has been investing in mindfulness to help employees focus and make more informed decisions by considering a wider array of options and to inspire creativity by fostering time to think (Schaufenbuel 2015). Indeed, there is mounting evidence for the benefits of pursuing a balanced lifestyle, including time off and meditation (Jabr 2013).

Aetna recently launched a mindfulness program for its 50,000 employees after a pilot clinical trial demonstrated a potential annual savings of $5,000 per employee through diminished health care costs and increased productivity (Achor and Gielan 2015). Aetna's chief executive officer Mark Bertolini recently appointed a chief mindfulness officer for the company and intends to take lessons Aetna has learned from its employee mindfulness programs to provide improved services to all of its 22 million members. These lessons include how to deliver mindfulness programs in scale via online tools (Achor and Gielan 2015).

At Google, one of the most sought-after internal courses, "Search Inside Yourself," focuses on mindfulness and teaches students to listen more not only to themselves but also to their coworkers. Many employees credit the course with improving their own productivity and interpersonal work relationships. Google is a cosponsor of the Wisdom 2.0 conference in San Francisco, a meeting for those who want to explore how "not only [to] live connected to one another through technology, but to do so in ways that are beneficial to our own well-being, effective in our work, and useful to the world" (Wisdom 2.0, 2015). The attraction of today's leading technology corporations to mindfulness may attest to the recognition that mindfulness provides a grounding needed for innovation. This grounding serves as a counterpoint to society's hyperconnectivity, which promises to quickly exceed that of our currently smartphone-connected society.

Moving beyond the smartphone, the mobile and Internet-based technologies appear to be converging on a far larger and more powerful set of smart connected devices. It is predicted that this Internet of Things (IoT), a network of devices, vehicles, buildings, and other objects embedded with electronic sensors, software, and connectivity components, will rapidly proliferate in the next few years. Fifty billion smart connected devices that will be communicating with each other are expected by 2020 (Iyer 2016). It is anticipated that the sensors and connectivity of the IoT will allow the gathering and analysis of information about ourselves and our environment on a scale never before possible. An example of a new type of data that can be gathered by even relatively old sensor technology is the demonstration by researchers at the Massachusetts Institute of Technology that they could reliably determine an individual's pulse from a videorecording of his or her face, by analyzing otherwise invisible changes in skin color that occur with each heartbeat (Wu et al. 2012). This means that whether individuals wear devices or simply inhabit environments with ambient sensors, the collection of an unprecedented set of data about their behavior and physiological state seems inevitable.

These new streams of data created by the IoT will invite technologists to develop tools to help increase our productivity. In addition, if there is interest, the expanding IoT can also be used to create tools to support a mindful existence—by increasing our understanding of ourselves and others through increased awareness and by boosting our appreciation of our global connectedness. There has been much publicity surrounding the need to protect the privacy of the data that the IoT collects (Porter and Heppelmann 2014). Care should also be taken to protect and support the mindfulness of the experiences that these new technologies create. A mindful approach to the development and use of the next generation of devices will be necessary to allow us to use them for our holistic benefit.

Key Points for Further Study and Reflection

- The recent widespread adoption of modern technology, despite its rich offering for humankind, has the potential to compromise our mindfulness.
- Mindfulness can be used to mediate our relationship with technology. Common technologies, including a phone, the Internet, and a car, can be used in such a way that they promote mindfulness.
- Technology has increased the accessibility of mindfulness resources and provided mobile applications and devices that can facilitate mindfulness. The efficacy of these apps and devices has yet to be demonstrated in large clinical trials.
- Mindfulness is being used to help improve employees' productivity and well-being. Mindfulness can play an even more important role amid the increasingly hyperconnectedness of the modern world.

TABLE 11–1. Technological tools for promoting mindfulness

Name	Developer (year if applicable)	Free to access?	Description	Web site
Online resources to promote mindfulness				
MBSR online course via Sounds True	University of Massachusetts Center for Mindfulness	No	The Stress Reduction Clinic at the University of Massachusetts offers an 8-week online training program consisting of self-guided videos; there is the opportunity to receive continuing education credits.	http://www.umassmed.edu/cfm/stress-reduction/mbsr-online/
Mindful	Mindful	Yes	Mindful publishes videos and the bimonthly *Mindful* magazine and organizes conferences. Mindful seeks to become a place to go for "insight, information, and inspiration to help us all live more mindfully." Its board of advisers includes Jon Kabat-Zinn	http://www.mindful.org
Mindful awareness practices (MAPs)	UCLA Mindful Awareness Research Center	No	University of California, Los Angeles offers an interactive online course that includes lectures, practice, and group feedback and discussion among 30–40 students	http://marc.ucla.edu/body.cfm?id=112
Mindfulness resources	University of Wisconsin Department of Family Medicine and Community Health	Yes	University of Wisconsin collated a variety of teaching modules, Web sites, books, audio resources, and online courses for patients interested in learning about mindfulness	http://www.fammed.wisc.edu/mindfulness/resources/
Stress Free Now	Cleveland Clinic Wellness Enterprise (2015)	Yes	Stress Free Now is a 6-week online course with a mobile application to reduce stress, increase positive emotions and energy, and teach practice relaxation techniques	http://www.clevelandclinicwellness.com/Programs/Pages/StressFreeNow.aspx

TABLE 11–1. Technological tools for promoting mindfulness *(continued)*

Name	Developer (year if applicable)	Free to access?	Description	Web site
Software applications to promote mindfulness				
Buddhify	Buddhify (2015)	Free trial, then paid	App that offers guided meditations for use while sitting at the desk, exercising, trying to get to sleep, or waiting in line at the grocery store, as well as a built-in timer for unguided meditations	http://buddhify.com
Calm	Calm (2016)	Free with paid in-app products	Software that offers calming imagery, music, and guidance to help users practice meditation whenever and wherever	http://www.calm.com
Headspace	Headspace (2014)	Free trial, then paid	App that allows users to choose session length, select specific areas of focus, and "buddy up with friends" for motivation	https://www.headspace.com
Mindfulness Daily	Inward Inc (2015)	No	App that allows users to set reminders to start daily meditations and track daily patterns and offers relaxing sounds and imagery to facilitate meditation	http://www.mindfulnessdailyapp.com
mSpot Meditation Finder	Damian Watson (2015)	Yes	App that provides information on and map views of locations for meditation, including parks, gardens, churches, piers, temples, and outdoor areas; users can contribute by sharing sites and rating and reviewing locations	http://mspot.info

TABLE 11–1. Technological tools for promoting mindfulness *(continued)*

Name	Developer (year if applicable)	Free to access?	Description	Web site
Software applications to promote mindfulness *(continued)*				
RescueTime	RescueTime (2008)	Free light version, then paid premium	Software that runs in the background of a computer or mobile device to track time spent on applications and Web sites, allowing users to keep track of how time is spent in a day, set alerts after a certain amount of time has been spent on a certain activity, and even block distracting Web sites	https://www.rescuetime.com
7 Second Meditation	Impressive Sounding, LLC (2015)	Yes	App that allows users to set timed reminders and push notifications to breathe, to reflect on life, or to be present	http://www.7secondmeditation.com
Smiling Mind	Smiling Mind (2015)	No	App and Web-based program offering age-appropriate guided meditations developed by a team of psychologists from Australia with expertise in youth and adolescent therapy; geared for age groups ranging from children as young as age 7 through adults	http://smilingmind.com.au
Stop, Breathe & Think	Tools for Peace (2014)	Yes	App that features a 5-minute program designed to develop and apply kindness and compassion by encouraging users to take a pause and check in, practice mindful breathing, and engage in meditation	http://stopbreathethink.org

TABLE 11–1. Technological tools for promoting mindfulness *(continued)*

Name	Developer (year if applicable)	Free to access?	Description	Web site
Devices to promote mindfulness				
Flex	Fitbit (2013)	No	A wrist-worn fitness and sleep monitor that tracks a user's activity and can alert the user who has been sedentary for too long	http://www.fitbit.com
Meaning to Pause	Meaning To Pause	No	A wristband that vibrates every 60 or 90 minutes to remind users to take the time to be more present	http://www.meaningtopause.com
Muse	Interaxon	No	A wearable headband-like device that purportedly detects user's state of mind and provides feedback on a mobile app to facilitate meditation	http://www.choosemuse.com
Prana	Prana	No	A wearable device that detects and tracks posture and breathing; it is synced with a mobile app that guides users through breathing techniques	http://prana.co
Shine 2	Misfit (2015)	No	A fitness and sleep monitor that is worn on the wrist or other wearable locations, tracks users' activity, and can alert users when they have been sedentary for too long; it is waterproof and requires no charging	http://www.misfit.com
Somadome	Somadome (2014)	No	A personal meditation pod that combines color immersion therapy and audiotherapy to help make any location a haven for meditation	http://www.somadome.com

TABLE 11–1. Technological tools for promoting mindfulness (*continued*)

Name	Developer (year if applicable)	Free to access?	Description	Web site
Devices to promote mindfulness (continued)				
Spire	Spire (2014)	No	A wearable device that detects breathing patterns and physical activity, correlates them to state of body and mind, and sends users messages to coach them into a "more calm, balanced state of mind"	https://www.spire.io
Thync	Thync	No	A wearable device worn over the side of the forehead and ear that purportedly uses brain stimulation to enhance mood; both stimulating and calming programs are available	http://www.thync.com

References

Achor S, Gielan M: The busier you are, the more you need mindfulness. Harv Bus Rev, December 18, 2015. Available at: https://hbr.org/2015/12/the-busier-you-are-the-more-you-need-mindfulness. Accessed January 16, 2016.

American Academy of Pediatrics: Media and Children. 2015. Available at: https://www.aap.org/en-us/advocacy-and-policy/aap-health-initiatives/pages/media-and-children.aspx. Accessed January 16, 2016.

Block JJ: Issues for DSM-V: Internet addiction. Am J Psychiatry 165(3):306–307, 2008 18316427

Boorstein S: Road Sage: Mindfulness Techniques for Drivers. Louisville, CO, Sounds True Publishing, 2006

Carissoli C, Villani D, Riva G: Does a meditation protocol supported by a mobile application help people reduce stress? Suggestions from a controlled pragmatic trial. Cyberpsychol Behav Soc Netw 18(1):46–53, 2015 25584730

Davis JM, Manley AR, Goldberg SB, et al: Mindfulness training for smokers via web-based video instruction with phone support: a prospective observational study. BMC Complement Altern Med 15:95, 2015 25886752

Gebel E: Getting past tense: dealing with stress the right way may safeguard your health. Diabetes Forecast 65(12):52–55, 2012 23270279

Giedd JN: The digital revolution and adolescent brain evolution. J Adolesc Health 51(2):101–105, 2012 22824439

Higgins S, Xiao Z, Katsipataki M: The Impact of Digital Technology on Learning: A Summary for the Education Endowment Foundation, School of Education, Durham University, Durham, UK, 2012

Howells A, Ivtzan I, Eiroa-Orosa F: Putting the "app" in happiness: a randomised controlled trial of a smartphone-based mindfulness intervention to enhance wellbeing. J Happiness Stud, October 2014, p 29

Isaacson W: Steve Jobs. New York, Simon & Schuster, 2015

Iyer B: To predict the trajectory of the Internet of Things, look to the software industry. Harv Bus Rev, February 25, 2016

Jabr F: Why your brain needs more downtime. Sci Am, October 15, 2013. Available at: http://www.scientificamerican.com/article/mental-downtime/. Accessed April 14, 2016.

Khoury B, Lecomte T, Fortin G, et al: Mindfulness-based therapy: a comprehensive meta-analysis. Clin Psychol Rev 33(6):763–771, 2013 23796855

Lam LT: Risk factors of Internet addiction and the health effect of Internet addiction on adolescents: a systematic review of longitudinal and prospective studies. Curr Psychiatry Rep 16(11):508, 2014 25212714

Lenhart A: Teens, smartphones & texting. Washington, DC, Pew Research Center, March 9, 2012. Available at: http://www.pewinternet.org/2012/03/19/teens-smartphones-texting/. Accessed January 10, 2016.

Lenhart A: Teens, social media & technology overview 2015. Washington, DC, Pew Research Center, April 9, 2015. Available at: http://www.pewinternet.org/2015/04/09/teens-social-media-technology-2015/. Accessed January 10, 2016.

Mani M, Kavanagh DJ, Hides L, Stoyanov SR: Review and evaluation of mindfulness-based iPhone apps. JMIR Mhealth Uhealth 3(3):e82, 2015 26290327

Moreno MA, Jelenchick L, Cox E, et al: Problematic Internet use among U.S. youth: a systematic review. Arch Pediatr Adolesc Med 165(9):797–805, 2011 21536950

Nhat Hanh T: Present Moment, Wonderful Moment: Mindfulness Verses for Daily Living. Berkeley, CA, Parallax Press, 2006

Nhat Hanh T: Dharma talk: the horse is technology. The Mindfulness Bell, November 10, 2013. Available at: http://static1.squarespace.com/static/55beacc8e4b0c17151842dbc/t/56be51de59827e9a672564cb/1455313379138/mb66.pdf. Accessed June 28, 2016.

Nhat Hanh T: Telephone Meditation. Buddhism Now. May 3, 2014. Available at: https://buddhismnow.com/2014/05/03/telephone-meditation-by-thich-nhat-hanh/. Accessed January 12, 2016.

Nielsen: The Total Audience Report: Q3 2015. December 10, 2015. Available at: http://www.nielsen.com/us/en/insights/reports/2015/the-total-audience-report-q3-2015.html. Accessed January 10, 2016.

Osbaldiston N (ed): Culture of the Slow: Social Deceleration in an Accelerated World. Basingstoke, UK, Palgrave Macmillan, 2013

Plaza I, Demarzo MMP, Herrera-Mercadal P, García-Campayo J: Mindfulness-based mobile applications: literature review and analysis of current features. JMIR Mhealth Uhealth 1(2):e24, 2013 25099314

Porter ME, Heppelmann JE: How smart, connected products are transforming competition. Harv Bus Rev, November 2014. Available at: https://hbr.org/2014/11/how-smart-connected-products-are-transforming-competition/ar/pr. Accessed July 19 2016.

Purcell K, Rainie L: Technology's Impact on Workers. Washington, DC, Pew Research Center, December 30, 2014. http://www.pewinternet.org/files/2014/12/PI_Web25WorkTech_12.30.141.pdf. Accessed January 10, 2016.

Rideout VJ, Foehr UG, Roberts DF: Generation M2: Media in the Lives of 8- to 18-Year-Olds. Menlo Park, CA, Kaiser Family Foundation, January 2010. Available at: https://kaiserfamilyfoundation.files.wordpress.com/2013/01/8010.pdf. Accessed April 14, 2016.

Schaufenbuel K: Why Google, Target, and General Mills are investing in mindfulness. Harv Bus Rev December 28, 2015. Available at: https://hbr.org/2015/12/why-google-target-and-general-mills-are-investing-in-mindfulness. Accessed July 19, 2016.

Smith A: U.S. Smartphone Use in 2015. Washington, DC, Pew Research Center, April 1, 2015. Available at: http://www.pewinternet.org/files/2015/03/PI_Smartphones_0401151.pdf. Accessed January 10, 2016.

Strasburger VC, Jordan AB, Donnerstein E: Health effects of media on children and adolescents. Pediatrics 125(4):756–767, 2010 20194281

UCLA Mindful Awareness Research Center: MAPs Class Schedule. Available at: http://marc.ucla.edu/body.cfm?id=85#mapsi-online. Accessed December 31, 2015.

Uhls YT, Michikyan M, Morris J, et al: Five days at outdoor education camp without screens improves preteen skills with nonverbal emotion cues. Comput Human Behav 39:387–392, 2014

Wisdom 2.0: Wisdom 2.0 Conference—Living with Awareness, Wisdom, and Compassion. 2015. Available at: http://www.wisdom2summit.com/. Accessed December 31, 2015.

Wu H, Rubinstein R, Shih E, et al: Eulerian video magnification for revealing subtle changes in the world. ACM Transactions on Graphics 31(4), Article No 65, July 2012

Yu MC, Wu H, Lee MS, Hung YP: Multimedia-assisted Breathwalk-aware system. IEEE Trans Biomed Eng 59(12):3276–3282, 2012 23203771

Appendix A

Audio Guided Meditations

INCLUDED with this book are two audio guided meditations for your use. We hope these will be helpful for you. It is recommended you familiarize yourself with the audio recordings to help you discern the most appropriate use of these guided meditation tools for your patients. Similarly, your own practice of these exercises will help you to navigate with your patients through challenging terrain they may encounter while working with difficult emotions. A brief description of each recording is provided below.

The audio guided meditations can be accessed online by navigating to www.appi.org/Zerbo.

Mindfulness Meditation Exercise
Author/narrator: Cory Muscara
Length: 15:10
Description: This exercise is intended for clinicians and can also be used with patients in or out of session. It can be used by beginners or experienced meditators. In this meditation, Cory guides the listener to practice letting go of distractions in order to open to a nonjudgmental state of awareness.

Meditation on Difficult Emotions
Author/narrator: Jonathan Kaplan, Ph.D.
Length: 21:10
Description: This mindfulness exercise is intended for use with patients in session. In this meditation Jonathan guides the listener in identifying, accepting, and working with challenging emotions.

Appendix B

Mindfulness Resources

Hint, Reminder, and Resource for Practice

- STOP: Stop, Take a Breath, Observe, Proceed
- Commit to only 1 minute per day
- Accountability with a friend or a coach: http://www.coach.me

Meditations

- **Free guided meditations:** Link to free guided meditations offered by the UCLA Mindful Awareness Research Center: http://marc.ucla.edu/body.cfm?id=22
- **The Free Mindfulness Project:** growing collection of free, downloadable mindfulness meditation exercises: www.freemindfulness.org
- **One-Moment Meditation:** YouTube link, "How to Meditate in a Moment": https://www.youtube.com/watch?v=F6eFFCi12v8
- **Headspace App:** App (with modest monthly charge) for different meditations: https://www.headspace.com
- **Calm App:** App with mindfulness meditations: https://itunes.apple.com/us/app/calm-meditate-sleep-relax/id571800810?mt=8
- **Insight Timer App:** Free app that provides guided meditations, includes bells (if you want a timer to start and finish), and acts as a meditation community where you can see hundreds of other people meditating around the world: https://insighttimer.com
- **Jon Kabat-Zinn guided meditations:** http://www.mindfulnesscds.com
- **Sip and Om:** A plethora of guided meditations for those who find it hard to get started or keep a regular practice: https://www.sipandom.com

Books

- *Full Catastrophe Living: Using the Wisdom of Your Body and Mind to Face Stress, Pain, and Illness*, revised edition, by Jon Kabat-Zinn. New York, Bantam Books, 2013
- *Mindfulness: An Eight-Week Plan for Finding Peace in a Frantic World*, by Mark Williams and Danny Penman. New York, Rodale Books, 2012
- *A Mindfulness-Based Stress Reduction Workbook*, by Bob Stahl and Elisha Goldstein. Oakland, CA, New Harbinger, 2010
- *The Mindful Brain: Reflection and Attunement in the Cultivation of Well-Being*, by Daniel J. Siegel. New York, WW Norton, 2007
- *Mindfulness in Plain English*, by Bhante Gunaratana and Henepola Gunaratana. New York, Simon & Schuster, 2011
- *The Miracle of Mindfulness: The Classic Guide to Meditation by the World's Most Revered Master*, by Thich Nhat Hanh. New York, Random House, 2008
- *The Places That Scare You: A Guide to Fearlessness in Difficult Times*, by Pema Chodron. Boston, MA, Shambhala, 2001
- *Real Happiness: The Power of Meditation (a 28-Day Program)*, by Sharon Salzberg. New York, Workman, 2010
- *Search Inside Yourself: The Unexpected Path to Achieving Success, Happiness (and World Peace)*, by Chade-Meng Tan, Daniel Goleman, and Jon Kabat-Zinn. HarperOne, New York, 2012
- *When Things Fall Apart: Heart Advice for Difficult Times*, by Pema Chodron. Boston, MA, Shambhala, 1997
- *Wherever You Go, There You Are*, by Jon Kabat-Zinn. New York, Hachette Books, 2005
- *You Are Not Your Pain: Using Mindfulness to Relieve Pain, Reduce Stress, and Restore Well-Being—An Eight-Week Program*, by Vidyamala Burch and Danny Penman. New York, HarperOne, 2015

Podcasts and Audio

- Audio Dharma—an archive of Dharma talks given by Gil Fronsdal, Andrea Fella, and various guest speakers at the Insight Meditation Center in California: http://audiodharma.org
- Sounds True—a Web site with a wealth of video and audio programs (many free) on mindfulness, meditation, and much more: www.soundstrue.com/store/

- Ellen Langer—Science of Mindlessness and Mindfulness: www.onbeing.org/program/ellen-langer-science-of-mindlessness-and-mindfulness/6332
- Weekly podcast at UCLA's Hammer Museum hosted by Diana Winston, Director of Mindfulness Education at the UCLA Mindful Awareness Research Center: http://marc.ucla.edu/body.cfm?id=107

Web Sites

- Mindful.org: the Web site for the magazine *Mindful*, which provides an assortment of articles and tips to help you live a mindful life
- Goamra.org: the Web site for the American Mindfulness Research Association, which serves as a professional resource for mindfulness research and provides information about current research efforts and local mindfulness training programs
- Dharmaseed.org: focuses on Western Buddhist *vipassanā* teachings; has many free talks and information about teachers and retreats
- Thehealingmind.org: the Web site for Dr. Marty Rossman's work in mind/body self-healing techniques; his approach focuses on guided imagery
- Drrogerwalsh.com: the Web site of Dr. Roger Walsh, Professor at the University of California at Irvine, with a lot of resources—articles, video talks, guided meditations, interviews
- Tarabrach.com: the Web site of respected teacher Tara Brach, with an abundance of resources, including free talks, meditations, and recommended readings
- Pocketmindfulness.com: a popular blog by Alfred James, a mindfulness coach and author

Videos

- Mindfulness with Jon Kabat-Zinn (Google Talk): https://www.youtube.com/watch?v=3nwwKbM_vJc
- Scientific power of meditation (short clip about the science of meditation): https://www.youtube.com/watch?v=Aw71zanwMnY
- Neuroscience of meditation with neuroscientist Richard Davidson (GoogleTechTalk): https://www.youtube.com/watch?v=7tRdDqXgsJ0

Articles

Harvard Business Review

- Mindfulness in the Age of Complexity (an interview with Ellen Langer), by Alison Beard: https://hbr.org/2014/03/mindfulness-in-the-age-of-complexity
- Mindfulness Can Literally Change Your Brain, by Christina Congleton, Britta K. Hölzel, and Sara W. Lazar: https://hbr.org/2015/01/mindfulness-can-literally-change-your-brain
- Mindfulness for People Who Are Too Busy to Meditate, by Maria Gonzalez: https://hbr.org/2014/03/mindfulness-for-people-who-are-too-busy-to-meditate

Retreat Centers Offering Mindfulness-Based Programs (Partial List)

- Esalen Institute, Big Sur, California: www.esalen.org
- Insight Meditation Society Retreat Center, Barre, Massachusetts: www.dharma.org
- Kripalu Center for Yoga & Health, Stockbridge, Massachusetts: www.kripalu.org
- Omega Institute, Rhinebeck, New York: www.eomega.org
- Shambhala Mountain Center, Red Feather Lakes, Colorado: www.shambhalamountain.org
- Spirit Rock Meditation Center, Woodacre, California: www.spiritrock.org
- Online resource to find local retreats: www.retreatfinder.com

Index

Page numbers printed in **boldface** type refer to tables or figures.

Acceptance, 29, 95
Acceptance and commitment therapy
 (ACT)
 examples of, 142–143
 for teaching mindful eating, 153
 for treatment of substance use
  disorders, 138–139, 141–143
Accomplishment/achievement, 116–117
 self-control and, 116
ACT. *See* Acceptance and commitment
 therapy
Actions, 72
Addictive disorders
 mindfulness-based intervention for,
  89–90
ADHD (attention-deficit/hyperactivity
 disorder)
 mindfulness-based intervention for, 88
Adolescents
 Kaplan's description of, 127
 mindfulness in, 126–128
 promoting mindfulness in, 121–133
  benefits of, 124–125
  impact, 124–125
  overview, 123–124
 risky behaviors and, 127–128
 smartphones and, 165
Aetna, mindfulness program, 172
Affect tolerance, 48
Allostasis, 11
Allostatic load/overload, 11
Allowing, 68
ANS (autonomic nervous system), 11
 regulation of, 12
Anxiety
 decreased levels with mindfulness, 17
 meditating and, 36
 mindfulness and, 11
 mindfulness-based intervention for,
  86–87

Attention
 control of, 92, 95, **93**
 enhanced, 47
 relaxation and, 14
 skills for, 27
Attention-deficit/hyperactivity disorder
 (ADHD)
 mindfulness-based intervention for, 88
Attitude
 nonjudgmental, 29
 nonstriving, 29
Autonomic nervous system (ANS), 11
 regulation of, 12
Aversion
 clinician, 56–57

Bare attention, 4
Beginner's mind, 29
Behavior
 influence of mindfulness on eating
  behaviors, 150–152
Binge-eating disorder
 in DSM-5, 149
Body
 mindfulness of, 34–35
 as mode of mindfulness, 15
 self-awareness of, 15–16
Boredom
 of the clinician, 55
Brain
 gray matter, 125
 mindfulness and, 13–14, 20
 prefrontal cortex, 12
 self-transcendence and, 18–20
 "wear and tear" on, 11
Breath
 mindfulness of, 33–34
Broaden-and-build theory, 108
Buddhify software application, **175**
Burnout of the clinician, 48

Calm software application, **175**
Car, 168–169
Case examples
    of mindfulness, 66, 69
    of problem formulation approach,
        96–97
CBT (cognitive-behavioral therapy)
    in youth, 131
Children
    description of child's mind, 129
    early childhood characterization, 126
    mindfulness in, 125–126
        exercises for, 129
    promoting mindfulness in, 121–133
        benefits of, 124–125
        impact, 124–125
        mindfulness training, 126
        overview, 123–124
        psychopathology and, 131–132
        working with children and
            mindfulness, 129–131
            consistency and routine with,
                129–130
Clinician, 45–59
    benefits of mindfulness for, 47–48
        attitudes and therapeutic presence,
            47–48
        reduction of burnout, 48
    boredom of, 55
    burnout of, 48
    challenges and barriers for clinician
        mindfulness, 53–58
        aversion, 56–57
        clinician barriers, 54–55
        compassion, 54–55
        doubt, 56
        restlessness and boredom, 55
        sensory craving, 56
        shifting from doing to being, 55
        sleepiness, 55–56
    establishing a mindfulness practice,
        49–53
        formal practice, 49–50
            attending retreats, 50
            establishing a daily practice, 49

finding a teacher, 50
            joining a community, 50
            training program, 49
        informal practice, 51–53
            communicating mindfully,
                52–53
            grounding practice, 51
            single tasking, 53
            sitting in silence with the
                patient, 51–52
        incorporating mindful eating in
            clinical practice, 156–159
        loving-kindness instruction, 57–58
        MBIs for treatment of substance use
            disorders, 144
Clock, 167
Cognitive-behavioral therapy (CBT)
    in youth, 131
Communication
    between clinician and patient, 52
Community
    clinician and, 50
Compassion meditation practice, 43
    benefits and by-products of, 43
    challenges to, 42
    clinician and, 54–55
    description of, 48
    meditation and, 40–43
    overview, 27
Concentration power, 27
Cravings
    examples of, 140–141
    with substance abuse disorders, 139–
        140
Csikszentmihályi, Mihály
    engagement and, 110–111

Dalai Lama, 121
Davidson, Richard
    studies with monks and meditation,
        124–125
DBT. *See* Dialectical Behavior Therapy
Depression
    mindfulness-based intervention for,
        82, 85–86

Dialectical Behavior Therapy (DBT), 11
for teaching mindful eating, 153
for treatment of substance use
disorders, 143
"Dose response," 124
Doubt
of the clinician, 56
DSM-5
binge-eating disorder in, 149

Eating disorders. *See also* Overeating
DBT and, 153
influence of mindfulness on, 150–152
mindfulness-based intervention for, 89
EEG. *See* Electroencephalogram
Electroencephalogram (EEG)
following a meditation program, 109
mindfulness and patterns of, 12
studies, 13
E-mail, 168
Emotional intelligence, 47
Emotions, 73
regulation of, 95–96, **93**
Empathy, 48
Engagement, 110–113
Csikszentmihályi and, 110–111
yoga and, 112–113
Epstein, Ronald M., 45
Equanimity, 27, 48
Eudaimonia
meaning and, 115
Eudaimonic turn, 105
External eating, 154

Fitbit Flex, 171
Flex
device to promote mindfulness, **177**
Flow
achievement of, 110–111
junk flow, 111
mindfulness meditation and, 111
music and, 112
Formal practice
description of, 30
establishing, 49–53

versus informal practice, 30–31
mindfulness outside of sessions, 74–
75
starting, 27*n*1, 31–32
Frankl, Victor
positive psychology and, 117
Free association
mindfulness and, 13

GATES (Goals, Actions, Thoughts,
Emotions, Senses), 72–73
Goals, 72
description of, 116
Goals, Actions, Thoughts, Emotions,
Senses (GATES), 72–73
Goldstein, Joseph
on karma, 6
Google
mindfulness program for, 172
Grounding
clinician and, 51

Hatha yoga, 21, 55, **83**
Headspace, 170–171
Headspace software application, **175**
Hedonism
meaning and, 115
Hindu technique, 5
Hippocrates, 147

Informal practice
description of, 30–31
establishing, 51–53
versus formal practice, 30–31
mindfulness outside of sessions, 76
Insight meditation, 3
Insight Meditation Society (IMS), 4
Intention
description of, 116–117
Internet
negative effects of, 166
positive use of, 168
Internet of Things (IoT), 173
Interoception, 106
IoT (Internet of Things), 173

Jobs, Steve, 163
Junk flow, 111

Kabat-Zinn, Jon, 79
    on mindful eating practice, 150
    on mindfulness, 3
    Mindfulness-Based Stress Reduction
        program, 4
Kaplan, Louise J.
    description of adolescents, 127
Karma
    Goldstein on, 6
Kindness, 17–18
    limbic system and, 16–18
    as mode of mindfulness, 15
    practice of, 20
Knowing, 68

Labeling, 35
Letting go, 29–30
Limbic system
    neuroscience and, 16–18
Linehan, Marsha M., 135
Listening
    mindful, 52, 53
LKM. *See* Loving-kindness meditation
Loving-kindness meditation (LKM), 107
    Fredrickson and, 108–109
    versus mindfulness-based stress
        reduction, 109
Loving-kindness practice, 38–40, 43
    benefits and by-products of, 43
    challenges to, 42
    instruction, 57–58
    limbic system and, 18
    as mode of mindfulness, 15
    overview, 27
    practice of, 20

MAPs (mindful awareness practices)
    online resource, **174**
MBCT. *See* Mindfulness-Based
    Cognitive Therapy

MB-EAT, 89. *See* Mindfulness-Based
    Eating Awareness Training;
    Mindfulness-Based Relapse Eating
    Awareness Training
MBI. *See* Mindfulness-based
    intervention
MBRP. *See* Mindfulness-Based Relapse
    Prevention
MBSR. *See* Mindfulness-Based Stress
    Reduction program
Meaning, 115–116
    eudaimonia and, 115
    hedonism and, 115
Meaning to Pause wristband, 171
    device to promote mindfulness, **177**
Medawi, 4
Meditation, 183
    as an integrative practice, 12
    audio guided, 181
    Davidson's studies with monks and,
        124–125
    "dose response," 124
    posture, 31–32
    relaxation response and, 11
    wellness and, 103–120
Memory, 17
Metacognition, 106
Mindful
    online resource, **174**
Mindful awareness practices (MAPs)
    online resource, **174**
Mindful eating, 147–161
    challenges in implementing, 159–160
    current protocols for teaching mindful
        eating, 153
    dysregulation theories of overeating,
        151
    external eating, 154
    externality theory of overeating,
        151–152
    history of mindful eating practice, 150
    incorporating in clinical practice,
        156–159

interventions, 152
Kabat-Zinn and, 150
mindful eating practices, **150**
overview, 149
psychosomatic theories of
    overeating, 151
research, 153–156
sample script for, **158**
Mindfulness
Aetna program for, 172
as an intervention in the treatment of
    psychopathology, 79–102
    anxiety disorders, 86–87
    attention-deficit/hyperactivity
        disorder, 88
    characteristics of mindfulness-
        based interventions, **83–84**
    for depression and suicidality, 82,
        85–86
    eating disorders, 89
    future directions, 98–99
    overview, 81
    personalized mindfulness-based
        treatment, 91–98
        emotion regulation, 95–96
        factors of therapeutic change,
            92, 95, **93–94**
        overview, 91–92
        primary mechanisms of change
            and treatment plan, 97–98
        problem formulation
            approach, 96–97
    psychosis, 90–91
    substance-related and addictive
        disorders, 89–90
    trauma and stress-related
        disorders, 87
articles, 186
books, 184
brain and, 11, 12, 13–14, 20
Buddha and, 3, 4
case examples of, 66, 69
    of problem formulation approach,
        96–97

definition of, 3
description of, 3, 27
free association and, 13
future of neuropsychiatry and, 20
Google program for, 172
history of, 1–7
impact on relationships, 114
influence on eating behaviors, 150–
    152
kindness and, 17–18
meditation and flow, 111
mindful eating, 147–161
modern roots of, 3–4
modes of, 15, 21
neuroscience of, 9–24
    integration of body and self-
        awareness, 15–16
    integration of mindfulness and
        psychotherapy, 13–14
    limbic system and, 16–18
    neocortex and, 15–16
    spectrum of, 15
PERMA and, 106
podcasts and audio, 184–185
in practice, 61–78
    conceptual overview of, 67–69
        allowing, 68
        knowing, 69
        perceiving, 67–68
        reflecting, 68–69
        stopping/slowing down, 67
    "fit" of, 63–66
        person, 65–66
        practice, 64–65
        purpose, 63–64
    improving ability to lead, 73–74
    inside of sessions, 69–72
        formal exercises, 69–70, 72
        informal exercises, 72–73
    obstacles, 76–77
    outside of sessions, 74–76
        formal practice, 74–75
        informal practice, 76
    overview, 63

Mindfulness *(continued)*
  in practice *(continued)*
    revisiting effectiveness of
      mindfulness, 77
    sample script for mindfulness of
      difficult emotions, **70–71**
    SPARK model, 67–69
  practice of, 25–44
    attention skills, 27
    attitudinal qualities of, 28–30
    compassion meditation, 40–43
      benefits and by-products of, 43
      challenges to, 42
      helpful tips, 41–42
      overview, 27
    formal versus informal, 30–31
    helpful tips for, 41–42
    loving-kindness, 38–40
      benefits and by-products of, 43
      challenges to, 42
      overview, 27
    versus mindfulness itself, 27
    misperceptions of, 30
    open-monitoring, 36–38
      benefits and by-products of, 38
      challenges to, 37
      choiceless awareness, 36–37
      mindful presence, 37
      overview, 27
    overview, 27
    starting a formal practice, 31–32
      meditation posture, 31–32
      settling in, 32
      use of a timer, 32
    task-focused, 32–36
      mindfulness of the body, 34–35
      mindfulness of the breath, 33–
        34
      mindfulness of sound, 33
      overview, 27
  promoting in children and
    adolescents, 121–133
  resources, 183–186
  retreat centers, 186

  role in psychiatry, 11
  self-transcendence and, 18–20
  sensitivity and, 17–18
  technological tools for promoting
    mindfulness, **174–178**
  technology and, 163–180
  vertical integration and, 13
  videos, 185
  web sites, 185
  wellness and, 103–120
Mindfulness-Based Cognitive Therapy
  (MBCT), 11, 82, 85
  characteristics of, **83**
  mindfulness-directed tasks, 138
  neurocognitive benefits of, 137
  practicing, 138
  studies of, 110
  for teaching mindful eating, 153
Mindfulness-Based Eating Awareness
  Training (MB-EAT), 89
  for teaching mindful eating, 153
Mindfulness-based intervention (MBI)
  overview, 81
  for substance use disorder treatment,
    89–90, 135–146
Mindfulness-Based Relapse Eating
  Awareness Training (MB-EAT)
  characteristics of, **84**
Mindfulness-Based Relapse Prevention
  (MBRP)
  characteristics of, **83**
  for treatment of substance use
    disorders, 90, 143–144
Mindfulness-Based Stress Reduction
  (MBSR) program, 4, 11, 82
  characteristics of, **83**
  versus loving-kindness meditation,
    109
  online resource, **174**
  for teaching mindful eating, 153
Mindfulness Daily software application,
  175
"Mindfulness revolution," 63
Mindfulness-to-meaning theory, 115

Mindset
    autonomic stress reaction and, 20
    as mode of mindfulness, 15
Misfit Shine 2, 171
mSpot Meditation Finder software
    application, **175**
    device to promote mindfulness, **177**
Music
    flow and, 112

Nhat Hanh, Thich, 1, 159
    on technology, 166
Neocortex
    neuroscience and, 15–16
Neuroplasticity, 11
Neuropsychiatry. *See also* Psychiatry;
    Psychopathology
    future of, 20
Neuroscience
    of mindfulness, 9–24
Noting, 35

Open-monitoring practice, 43
    benefits and by-products of, 38
    challenges to, 37
    choiceless awareness, 36–37
    mindful presence, 37
    overview, 27
    starting, 36–38
Overeating. *See also* Eating disorders
    dysregulation theories of, 151
    externality theory of, 151–152
    psychosomatic theories of, 151
    research, 154

Panic attacks, 96–97
    mindfulness during, 97–98
Patience, 29
PBCT. *See* Person-Based Cognitive
    Therapy
PERMA (Positive emotions, Engagement,
    [positive] relationships, Meaning/
    purpose, and Accomplishment/
    achievement), 106, 118

Person-Based Cognitive Therapy (PBCT)
    characteristics of, **84**
    for psychosis, 91
Peterson, Christopher
    positive relationships and, 113
PFC (prefrontal cortex), 12
Phone, 167–168
    cell phone use, 168
    smartphones and adolescents, 165
Positive emotions, 107–110
    description of, 107
    studies of, 107–110
Positive relationships, 113–115
    Peterson and, 113
Posttraumatic stress disorder (PTSD)
    mindfulness-based intervention for, 87
Prana
    device to promote mindfulness, **177**
Prefrontal cortex (PFC), 12
Proprioception, 106
Psychiatry. *See also* Neuropsychiatry;
    Psychopathology
    role of mindfulness in, 11
Psychology. *See also* Psychopathology
    definition of, 117–118
    positive, 117
Psychopathology. *See also* Psychiatry
    cognitive-behavioral therapy and, 131
    mindfulness and, 131–132
Psychosis
    mindfulness-based intervention for,
        90–91
PTSD (posttraumatic stress disorder)
    mindfulness-based intervention for, 87

RAIN (Recognize, Accept, Investigate,
    and Nonidentify), 67n1
    elements of, **157**
    for mindful eating in clinical
        practice, 156
Reflecting, 68
Relaxation
    attention and, 14
Rescue Time, 168

Rescue Time software application, **176**
Restlessness
    clinician, 55
Retreats
    clinician and, 50

Schizophrenia spectrum disorders
    mindfulness-based intervention for, 90
Scripts
    for mindful eating, **158**
    for mindfulness of difficult emotions,
        70–71
Self
    compassion and, 54
Self-awareness, 96, **93–94**
    of the body, 15–16
    default mode network and, 16
    integration of body and, 15–16
    meta-awareness, 96
    self-compassion, 18, 96
Self-compassion, 18, 96
Self-control
    accomplishment/achievement and, 116
Self-regulation
    limbic system and, 16–18
Self-transcendence
    mindfulness and, 18–20
Seligman, Martin, 105
Senses, 73
Sensitivity, 17–18
    limbic system and, 16–18
    as mode of mindfulness, 15
    practice of, 20
Sensory clarity, 27
Sensory craving
    clinician, 56
7 Second Meditation software
    application, **176**
Shame
    examples of, 139
    with substance abuse disorders, 139
SHINE (Stroke Hyperglycemia Insulin
    Network Effort), 155
Shine 2
    device to promote mindfulness, **177**

Siegel, Daniel, 9
Silence
    clinician and patient, 51–52
Single tasking
    clinician, 53
Sleep
    EEG studies and, 13
Sleepiness
    clinician, 55–56
Smiling Mind software application, **176**
Social connectedness, 47
Somadome
    device to promote mindfulness, **177**
Sound
    mindfulness of, 33
SPARK model, 67–69, 78
Speaking
    mindful, 52–53
Spire device to promote mindfulness,
    178
Stop, Breathe & Think software
    application, **176**
Stress Free Now
    online resource, **174**
Stress-related disorders
    mindfulness-based intervention for, 87
Substance use disorders (SUDs)
    acceptance and commitment therapy,
        138–139
    mechanism of action, 137–138
    mindfulness-based interventions for,
        89–90, 135–146
    acceptance and commitment
        therapy, 141–143
    clinicians treating SUDs, 144
    cravings, 139–141
    dialectical behavioral therapy, 143
    mindfulness-based relapse
        prevention, 143–144
    overview, 141
    relapse, 138–139
    shame, 139
    12-step literature, 144
SUDs. *See* Substance use disorders
Suicidality

mindfulness-based intervention for, 82, 85–86

Task-focused practice, 43
  benefits and by-products of, 35–36
  challenges to, 36
  mindfulness of the body, 34–35
  mindfulness of the breath, 33–34
  mindfulness of sound, 33
  overview, 27
  starting, 32–36
Technology
  adoption of, 173
  facilitating access to mindfulness
      resources, 170
  mindfulness and, 163–180
    future directions of, 172–173
    overview, 165
  mindfulness-related devices, 171–172
  mobile applications supporting
      mindfulness, 170–171
  Nhat Hanh on, 166
  for promoting mindfulness, 169–172
    mobile applications supporting
        mindfulness, 170–171
    overview, 169–170
    technology facilitating access to
        mindfulness resources, 170
  taking a break from, 166
  technological tools for promoting
      mindfulness, **174–178**
  tools for promoting mindfulness,
      174–178
  using mindfully, 165–169

car, 168–169
clock, 167
Internet, 168
mindfulness-related devices, 171–
    172
phone, 167–168
Thoreau, Henry David, 61
Thoughts, 72–73
Thync, 171
  device to promote mindfulness, **178**
Timer, 32
TM (transcendental meditation), 5
Transcendental Meditation (TM), 5
Trauma disorders
  mindfulness-based intervention for, 87
Trust, 29
12-step-based interventions, 144

Values
  clarification of, 96
von Goethe, Johann Wolfgang, 103

Watts, Alan, 25
Well-being
  measurement of, 106

Yoga, 21, 55, 76, 112–113, 114, 123, **83,
    84, 93, 95,**
  engagement and, 112–113

Zen meditation, 5, 21
  followers of, 5